Paula Torrano Belmonte
Lydia Fructuoso González

Antifungal therapy in the hematologic patient

Paula Torrano Belmonte
Lydia Fructuoso González

Antifungal therapy in the hematologic patient

Systematic review on antifungal therapy indicated in hematopoietic stem cell transplantation

ScienciaScripts

Cover image: www.ingimage.com

This book is a translation from the original published under ISBN 978-620-2-24627-9.

Publisher:
Sciencia Scripts
is a trademark of
Dodo Books Indian Ocean Ltd. and OmniScriptum S.R.L publishing group

120 High Road, East Finchley, London, N2 9ED, United Kingdom
Str. Armeneasca 28/1, office 1, Chisinau MD-2012, Republic of Moldova, Europe
Managing Directors: Ieva Konstantinova, Victoria Ursu
info@omniscriptum.com

Printed at: see last page
ISBN: 978-620-8-38624-5

Index

1. Abbreviations

AEMPS: Agencia Española del Medicamento y Productos Sanitarios

AI: aspergilosis invasiva

Alo-TPH: Trasplante alogénico

ASCO: American Society of Clinical Oncology
ATG: Inmunoglobulina antitimocitica

Auto-TPH: Trasplante autólogo

Cmáx: Concentraciones máximas

CMH: células madre hematopoyéticas

CMV : Citomegalovirus

CYP: Citocromos hepáticos

DMPC: L-α-dimiristoilfosfatidilcolina

DMPG: L-α-dimiristoilfosfatidilglicerol

ECIL: European Conference on Infections in Leukemia

EICH: Enfermedad injerto contra huésped

EMR: Enfermedad mínima residual

EORTC: European Organization for Research and Treatment of Cancer/Invasive Fungal Infections Cooperative Group

EPO: Eritropoyetina

FDA: Food and drug administration

G-CSF: factores estimulantes de colonias granulociticas

IDSA: Infectious Diseases Society of America

IFI: infección fúngica invasiva

LLA: leucemia linfoblástica aguda

MO: médula ósea

MSG: Infectious Diseases Mycoses Study Group

PABA: ácido para-aminobenzoico

PCR: Polimerase chain reaction

P-gp: Glicoproteina P

PH: progenitores hematopoyéticos

QC: Quimerismo completo

QM: Quimerismo mixto

SCU: sangre de cordón umbilical

SEIMC: Sociedad Española de Enfermedades Infecciosas y Microbiología

SIDA: Síndrome Inmunodeficiencia Humana

SMD: síndromes mielodisplásicos

SP: sangre periférica

TCMH:Trasplante de células madre hematopoyéticas

TPH: trasplante de progenitores hematopoyéticos

UGT: Uridina difosfato glucuronosiltransferasa

2. Summary

Fungal diseases are a type of disease associated with a patient undergoing hematopoietic stem cell transplantation (HSCT). HSCT is a therapy to replace a damaged hematopoietic system with a healthy one from a donor. Hematopoietic stem cells are those capable of regenerating all cell types of blood cells.

The aim of this review is to know the hematologic transplant patient and the characteristics that predispose him/her to suffer invasive fungal infections, as well as to know the methods of prophylaxis and treatment and to describe the most commonly used antifungal drugs.

For this purpose, a bibliographic search was carried out in different databases such as Pubmed, Cochrane Library and Science Direct, limiting the search to 10 years and English language. Initially, 1,113 articles were found, to which a series of inclusion and exclusion criteria were applied, to finally select 105 of them.

Patients undergoing these types of transplants are at risk of bacterial, viral and antifungal infections, especially during the period of neutropenia; therefore, it is essential to know the symptoms and management of symptoms in order to control infections and improve the prognosis of the graft.

Invasive fungal infection (IFI) caused by filamentous fungi is the most common fungal infection in individuals with hematologic diseases and hematopoietic stem cell transplantation with high morbidity and mortality. The main causative agent is the fungus *Aspergillus*. A critical assessment of the individual risk of IFI for each patient is important to select the best prophylactic and/or therapeutic approach to increase patient survival.

Risk factors for invasive aspergillosis are high patient age, graft versus host disease, immunosuppressive therapy, steroid use, neutropenia and some types of transplants such as umbilical cord transplants, T-cell depletion and incompatible allogeneic transplants.

Key words: antifungal therapy, hematopoietic transplantation, invasive fungal infection.

AEMPS: Agencia Española del Medicamento y Productos Sanitarios

AI: aspergilosis invasiva

Alo-TPH: Trasplante alogénico

ASCO: American Society of Clinical Oncology

ATG: Inmunoglobulina antitimocitica

Auto-TPH: Trasplante autólogo

Cmáx: Concentraciones máximas

CMH: células madre hematopoyéticas

CMV : Citomegalovirus

CYP: Citocromos hepáticos

DMPC: L-α-dimiristoilfosfatidilcolina

DMPG: L-α-dimiristoilfosfatidilglicerol

ECIL: European Conference on Infections in Leukemia

EICH: Enfermedad injerto contra huésped

EMR: Enfermedad mínima residual

EORTC: European Organization for Research and Treatment of Cancer/Invasive Fungal Infections Cooperative Group

EPO: Eritropoyetina

FDA: Food and drug administration

G-CSF: factores estimulantes de colonias granulociticas

IDSA: Infectious Diseases Society of America

IFI: infección fúngica invasiva

LLA: leucemia linfoblástica aguda

MO: médula ósea

MSG: Infectious Diseases Mycoses Study Group

PABA: ácido para-aminobenzoico

PCR: Polimerase chain reaction

P-gp: Glicoproteina P

PH: progenitores hematopoyéticos

QC: Quimerismo completo

QM: Quimerismo mixto

SCU: sangre de cordón umbilical

SEIMC: Sociedad Española de Enfermedades Infecciosas y Microbiología

SIDA: Síndrome Inmunodeficiencia Humana

SMD: síndromes mielodisplásicos

SP: sangre periférica

TCMH:Trasplante de células madre hematopoyéticas

TPH: trasplante de progenitores hematopoyéticos

UGT: Uridina difosfato glucuronosiltransferasa

Abstract

Fungal diseases are a type of diseases associated with patients undergoing hematopoietic stem cell transplantation (HSCT). HSCT is a replacement therapy of an altered hematopoietic system with a healthy one from a donor. Hematopoietic stem cells are those capable of regenerating all lineages of hematopoietic cells.

The objective of this review is to know about the hematological transplant patient and the characteristics that predispose him to suffer from invasive fungal infections, to learn the methods of prophylaxis and treatment and to describe the antifungal drugs used.

It was carried out a bibliographic research in different databases such as Pubmed, Cochrane Library and Science Direct, limiting the search to 10 years and English language. Initially, 1,113 articles were found, to which the inclusion and exclusion criteria were applied, finally selecting 105 of them.

Patients undergoing these types of transplants are at risk for bacterial, viral, and antifungal infections, especially during the period of neutropenia. That is why it is essential to know the symptoms and their management in order to control infections and improve the prognosis of the graft.

Invasive fungal infection (IFI) by filamentous fungi is the most common fungal infection in patients with hematological diseases and with hematopoietic stem cell transplantation with high morbidity and mortality. The main causative agent is the *Aspergillus*. A critical evaluation of the individual risk of IFI per patient, selecting the best prophylactic and/or therapeutic method is key to increase the survival of these patients.

Risk factors for invasive aspergillosis include patient age, graft-versus-host disease, immunosuppressive therapy, steroid use, neutropenia, and some types of transplants such as those from the umbilical cord, depletion of T cell and incompatible allogeneic transplants.

Keywords: antifungal therapy, hematopoietic transplant, invasive fungal infection.

3. Introduction

3.1. Hematopoietic stem cell transplantation

Hematopoietic progenitor transplantation (HSCT) or hematopoietic stem cell transplantation (HSCT) was introduced into the clinic in the 1950s and is currently maintained as a therapy capable of achieving disease-free survival for a large number of congenital and acquired pathologies. (1).

Currently, HSCT is used as a treatment for individuals with diseases affecting the bone marrow (congenital or acquired) and to rescue patients with hematologic diseases or certain types of cancer from the adverse effects caused by high doses of chemotherapy or radiotherapy. (2).

HSCT is a cell therapy in which the altered hematopoietic system is replaced by a healthy one in order to replace it so that it can develop normal hematopoiesis in the long term. Hematopoietic progenitors (HPCs) or hematopoietic stem cells (HSCs) are those capable of repopulating all hematopoietic cell lines when transplanted. HSCs can be obtained from bone marrow (BM), peripheral blood (PB) or umbilical cord blood (UCB). (1).

HSCT is used as a therapy to cure neoplastic and non-neoplastic hematological diseases, such as lymphomas, myelomas, leukemias, medullary aplasia, immunodeficiencies and congenital diseases of the hematopoietic system. HSCT can be allogeneic (Allo-HCT), if the donor of the progenitors is an individual different from the patient, and autologous or autogenic (Auto-HCT) if the donor and recipient are the same individual (1).

Donor selection must follow a series of requirements in order of importance: HLA compatibility between donor and recipient, cytomegalovirus serological status of donor and recipient, bone marrow as a source of progenitors, patient age (preferably young donor), donor gender (preferably male donor for male recipient), higher AB0 compatibility. (1).

Types of transplantation (1):

autologous HSCT

The patient's own stem cells are collected and cryopreserved for a few days or weeks before beginning the conditioning phase. Bone marrow progenitor procurement is rarely used and peripheral blood is preferred as a source.

The aim is to administer high doses of chemotherapy to kill the disease and subsequently infuse the patient's own progenitors, otherwise a life-threatening hematological aplasia may occur.

Autotransplantation is used as therapy for lymphoproliferative diseases, solid tumors and autoimmune diseases. However, for non-neoplastic congenital hemopathies and leukemias it does not seem to be effective.

allogeneic HSCT

The cells infused into the patient come from another donor. Because of this, there is a balance between the graft-versus-host effect and the graft-versus-recipient effect. The indications for allo-HCT are acute myeloid leukemia and myelodysplastic syndromes (MDS), acute lymphoblastic leukemia (ALL), lymphoproliferative syndromes and for non-neoplastic diseases, such as severe bone marrow aplasia and congenital immunodeficiencies.

HLA compatibility between donor and recipient is key, since an immune reaction occurs in both directions; on the one hand, the donor's progenitor cells are detected as foreign after infusion, and in the opposite direction, when the donor's cells recognize the recipient's tissues as foreign.

Donor selection:

The ideal donor is one with whom the recipient shares each of the 2 alleles of the five major loci, which is referred to as a 10/10 match and is considered the standard. Table 1 lists the five major HLA loci.

Histocompatibility is the most important factor for the success of Allo-TPH. An HLA-identical sibling is considered the best option, but if this is not possible, an unrelated but histocompatibly matched sibling donor is preferred.

Table 1. HLA locus

HLA CLASS I TYPING	HLA CLASS II TYPING
Locus HLA - A	HLA locus - DRB1
HLA - B locus	HLA Locus - DQB1
HLA - C Locus	

Sequence of transplantation processes:

1. Hematopoietic progenitor procurement

PH are obtained from the source of choice, either umbilical cord, bone marrow, or peripheral blood and cryopreserved, leaving them available for the date of engraftment to the recipient. To date, the most important factor in determining the quality of the engraftment is the CD34+ cell count. The CD34 receptor is found on the membrane of 1.4% of nucleated bone marrow cells. (3).

Graft manipulation

In this phase, ex vivo tumor cells are removed, CD34+ progenitors are selected, T lymphocytes are removed, red blood cells are reduced due to blood group incompatibility or the volumes initially obtained to be cryopreserved are reduced.

3. Conditioning

It is the combination of chemotherapy and radiotherapy that is infused to the patient days prior to the administration of the progenitors. The purpose of the conditioning is to eliminate the tumor cells, thus eliminating the underlying pathology, reaching a state of immunosuppression in order to be able to implant the graft and prevent the recipient's reaction against the donor. (1).

Depending on the chemotherapy and/or radiotherapy protocols used, conditioning regimens are termed myeloablative when they eradicate all stem cells from the bone marrow and non-myeloablative when they cause minimal cytopenia but significant lymphopenia.

In the case of autologous transplant conditioning, these consist of chemotherapy alone and in some cases also irradiation. However, in unrelated donor allogeneic transplant patients, the administration of antithymocyte globulin or alemtuzumab is necessary. (1).

PH infusion

This is the moment when the PH are thawed and administered to the patient. This day is considered day 0 of the transplant.

5. Post-transplant aplasia

Period of disappearance of the cells that occupy the marrow that the patient reaches after the infusion of the PH. Because of this state, the recipient requires care in hospital units dedicated to his care.

6. Prendimiento

It consists of the hematological recovery of the patient. It occurs between days 10-14 after PH infusion, when the patient's first cells appear (leukocytes, reticulocytes and platelets). When HSCT has been performed from peripheral blood PH, a faster recovery is achieved. (1).

7. Immune recovery

State achieved approximately 6 months after transplant infusion. T and B lymphocyte subpopulations appear and immunoglobulins are produced.

3.2.Complications of HSCT

Complications of HSCT are chronologically related. From the beginning of conditioning until days 14-28 after infusion of the progenitors, toxic complications associated with conditioning regimens, neutropenia and thrombocytopenia caused by the conditioning regimens may appear. The most important and serious complications are the infections that appear during the patient's neutropenia. The phase of bone marrow aplasia lasts between 2 and 4 weeks. In order to shorten the duration of neutropenia, administration of granulocyte colony stimulating factors (G-CSF) is recommended. Also, during this period, blood transfusions are usually very frequent.

In autologous transplantation, no serious complications are observed after delivery. Occasionally, secondary fever or infections caused by catheter or airway access may occur. In the case of allogeneic transplantation, the period occurring from the donor to day +100 post-transplantation is considered critical. Hematologic recovery requires between 6 and 12 months and the use of immunosuppressive treatment to avoid rejection puts these patients at greater risk of suffering opportunistic infections.

A. Complications of the conditioning process

Conditioning is a fundamental part of the transplantation process. It has two fundamental missions: anti-tumor activity and that of facilitating engraftment. It consists of a combination of chemotherapy, which may or may not be associated with radiotherapy. They are administered at high doses in defined schedules with respect to the day of infusion of hematopoietic progenitors (Day 0) (1). Table 2 lists some of the drugs used in the conditioning of HSCT (1).

Types of conditioning according to intensity:

- Myeloablative conditioning: This is the conventional conditioning regimen. It consists of the administration of high doses of radiotherapy and/or chemotherapy with alkylating agents. They have a maximum tumoricidal effect but are associated with high toxicity.

- Reduced intensity conditioning: consists of the administration of chemotherapy with lower doses; thus, better tolerance is achieved and to avoid rejection, the intensity of immunosuppression is increased. The toxicity that appears is lower.

- Non-myeloablative conditioning: causes minimal cytopenia and can be administered without PH infusion support.

Due to the drugs used in the conditioning phase, various types of toxicities appear, as shown in Table 3.

Table 2. Drugs in HSCT conditioning.

Pharmacological group		Drug	
Alkylating agents	Nitrogen mustards	Cyclophosphamide	ALO and AUTO
		Melphalan	AUTO and ALO
	Alkylsulfonate	Busulfan	ALO and AUTO
	Ethyleneamines	Tiotepa	ALO and AUTO
	Nitrosoureas	Carmustina	AUTO and ALO
	Platinums	Carboplatin	AUTO
Antimetabolites	Pyrimidine analogs	Cytarabine	ALO and AUTO
	Purine analogs	Fludarabine	ALO
Topoisomerase inhibitors		Etoposide	ALO and AUTO

Immunosuppressants		Antithymocyte immunoglobulin (ATG)	ALO

Table 3. Complications occurring in the HSCT patient due to conditioning regimens.

	Toxicity
Gastrointestinal	nausea and vomiting, diarrhea, mucositis, caloric balance
Cutaneous	Color changes, desquamation, dryness, alopecia
Hemorrhagic cystitis	Secondary to drugs (cyclophosphamide, busulfan or etoposide) or infections (polyomavirus, BK, adenovirus, CMV).
Other	Hepatic, cardiac, renal, pulmonary, neurologic

B. Neutropenia

Neutropenia is defined as an absolute neutrophil count less than 1,000 cells/µL, equivalent to 1.0×10^9 */L. Severe neutropenia* is known as neutrophil count less than 500 cells/µL (equivalent to $< 0.5 \times 10^9$ /L) and *profound neutropenia* as neutrophil count less than 100/µL (equivalent to $< 0.1 \times 10^9$ /L). Neutropenia is considered prolonged if it lasts longer than one week. Patients undergoing cytotoxic chemotherapy and HSCT are at risk for bacterial, viral, and antifungal infections, especially during the period of neutropenia (4).

Neutrophils are a critical part of the patient's defense, particularly against bacteria and fungi. The risk of infection increases as the severity of neutropenia increases and is considered maximal in those patients who experience profound and prolonged neutropenia just after aggressive chemotherapy, which occurs in the periods before HSCT engraftment and after chemotherapy for the treatment of acute leukemia (5). Prevention and proper management of neutropenia is important to avoid possible future complications, such as hypotension, renal and respiratory failure, septic shock or cardiac failure.

Fever in neutropenic patients is defined as a temperature above 38° C maintained for one hour. (5). Neutropenic fever occurs in at least 25-30% and mortality occurs in 11% of patients undergoing HSCT (6)(7). Risk factors for neutropenic fever should be systematically evaluated in patients, including the characteristics of the patient, the type of cancer and the implanted treatment.

C. Infections

In HSCT recipients, physicians face two problems: the high incidence of bacterial sepsis and the high mortality in case of Gram-negative bacterial infections. Additionally, in the absence of neutrophils, which are responsible for most clinical symptoms of bacterial infections (access, infiltrates, pyuria,...) fevers are the only presenting symptom in these cases. In addition, fevers are among the most non-specific symptoms and there are many more causes for which they can appear in a neutropenic patient, such as fungal infections, viral infections, drug reactions, transfusions, underlying diseases, graft syndromes, graft versus host disease, cytokine release syndrome, rejection and hemophagocytosis (1).

The most recommended antimicrobial prophylaxis in immunosuppressed patients according to the guidelines of the American Society of Clinical Oncology (ASCO) and the Infectious Diseases Society of America (IDSA) are as follows (5) (8) (9) (10):

- Antibiotic prophylaxis with quinolones is recommended in patients at high risk for neutropenic fever or severe neutropenia, especially more common in those patients with acute myeloid leukemia, myelodysplastic syndrome or HSCT treated with myeloablative chemotherapy regimens. (11) (12). Empiric antibiotic therapy begins with piperacillin- tazobactam, ceftazidime or cefepime and then the antibiotic is modified if necessary. With this strategy, carbapenems remain as a second line of treatment in those patients in whom initial therapy fails or the infection is maintained. Another strategy is to add an aminoglycoside to the beta-lactam. The empiric addition of vancomycin is not recommended unless the patient has symptoms of Gram-positive infection (13). Traditionally, the duration of antibiotic therapy was maintained until neutrophil counts recovered, with the intention of avoiding relapses. In the last decade, the guidelines proposed by the IDSA and European Conference on Infections in Leukemia (ECIL), antibiotic therapy could be stopped after 3 days or more of intravenous therapy in patients who have reached hemodynamic stability or in those who have been fever-free for more than 2 days, regardless of the granulocyte count or the expected duration of neutropenia (1). If despite antibiotic therapy, patients continue to maintain fever, there are necessary factors to consider. If there are no clear signs of clinical deterioration, and markers of inflammation are improving, it may be due to a slow response to treatment. Alternatively, non-bacterial infections, such as viral infections, or mucositis should be considered as reasons for worsening. In addition, galactomaman or other tests should be performed to rule out fungal infection. (14). If the patient's clinical condition deteriorates, it is recommended to repeat all tests, increase antibiotic coverage and start antifungal therapy (1). (1).

- Antifungal prophylaxis should be performed with an oral triazole or parenteral echinocandins in patients with neutropenia affected by acute myeloid leukemia, myelodysplastic syndrome or HSCT. Prophylaxis should be initiated while awaiting results confirming infection. This section will be developed later. Prophylaxis with trimethoprim and sulfamethoxazole is recommended in patients receiving chemotherapy regimens who have a greater than 3.5% risk of developing pneumonia caused by *Pneumocystis jirovecci*.

- Antiviral prophylaxis with acyclovir for patients with acute myeloid leukemia, myelodysplastic syndrome or HSCT is indicated in patients seropositive for herpes simplex virus. Prophylaxis with tenofovir or entecavir is recommended for patients at high risk of hepatitis B reactivation. (15).

- Annual vaccination against *influenza* virus with inactivated vaccines is recommended in all patients receiving chemotherapy for hematologic malignant syndromes. (16).

- Patients with neutropenia and receiving chemotherapy should avoid prolonged contact with environments that have a high concentration of fungal spores, such as construction, demolition or intensive gardening exposure.

D. Graft-versus-host disease (GVHD):

The most feared complication of allogeneic transplantation. Occurs when donor T cells recognize host cells as foreign. It can present in acute or chronic clinical form. The main difference is from the day they appear, i.e. before or after day +100 of infusion.

Acute GVHD (classified in four grades I, II, III and IV) occurs in 30-60% of patients and causes death in 20% of the cases. Acute GVHD can appear up to day +100 after transplantation, while delayed acute GVHD appears after +100. It mainly affects the skin causing maculopapular rash, the liver causing jaundice and the intestine causing diarrhea. The most relevant clinical manifestations of acute GVHD are listed in Table 4. The pathophysiology of acute GVHD is due to tissue injury by the conditioning process, which causes activation of host antigen presenting cells and activation of donor T cells, and finally, the effector phase by the release of proinflammatory cytokines and tissue necrosis. (17).

Immunosuppressive agents such as cyclosporine, trachrolimus, mycophenolate or methotrexate are used for prophylaxis of acute GVHD. For the treatment of grade I acute GVHD, which only affects the skin, topical corticosteroids can be used. More advanced grades of GVHD already need intravenous therapy, such as high doses of intravenous methylprednisolone. Striking the balance between treatment with immunosuppressants and maintaining infection control still remains a challenge. Second-line therapies include monoclonal antibodies such as alemtuzumab or infliximab, as well as JAK1 inhibitors such as ruxolitinib or vedolizumab. (1).

Table 4. Clinical Manifestations of Acute GVHD (1).

Organ	Clinical manifestations
Skin	Maculopapular erythematous rash (hands and soles of the feet). It may progress and affect the whole body, producing itching and pain. In severe cases, blistering and desquamation occur.

Liver	Cholestasis and elevation of cholestatic enzymes rather than transaminases.
Gastrointestinal tract	Anorexia, nausea and vomiting. Watery diarrhea, which in some cases may contain fresh blood and mucus, and may also be accompanied by paralytic ileus.

Chronic GVHD is the most relevant cause of death without recurrent or progressive disease after transplantation manifesting as multisystem involvement. It occurs in 20-40% of long-term survivors (18). Chronic involvement appears between 3 months and 2 years post-transplant. The classic clinical manifestations are autoimmune syndromes, such as myasthenia or myositis, but in general, it can affect any organ. Table 5 describes the most relevant clinical manifestations. The pathophysiology is due to alterations in the mechanisms of innate and specific immunity. (19). In addition to the damage it causes, chronic GVHD appears to have a protective role in the progression of malignant disease (19).

The first line of treatment is steroids alone or in combination with calcineurin inhibitors (cyclosporine or tacrolimus). Generally, first-line therapy achieves remission of chronic GVHD in approximately 20% of adult patients. If symptoms progress during the first 4 weeks of first-line therapy or there is no improvement of symptoms within about 12 weeks, then second-line therapy should be switched to second-line therapy. (1). As second-line therapy, no more than 3 immunosuppressive agents are recommended. Drugs such as imatinib and retinoids are recommended only in cases with symptoms of sclerosis. (1).

Table 5. Clinical manifestations of chronic GVHD (1)

Organ	Clinical manifestations

Skin	Maculopapular erythematous rash (hands and soles of feet), pruritus. Pigmentation alterations, papulosquamous lesions, ichthyosis, keratosis.
Eyes	Keratitis, atrophy of the lacrimal gland, dry eye syndrome, blepharitis, inflammation of the conjunctiva.
Oral mucosa	Erythema, ulcers, destruction of salivary glands, gingivitis, periodontitis, loss of teeth,
Liver	Cholestasis
Gastrointestinal tract	Dysphagia, nausea, vomiting, Chronic diarrhea and malabsorption syndrome
Genitalia	Vaginal dryness, ulcers.
Lung	Symptoms of progressive and irreversible obstruction, lymphocytic alveolitis, interstitial fibrosis.
Joints and muscles	Restriction of joint movements, rheumatic complications, sclerosis.

E. Rejection of the transplant:

Engraftment is defined by the first 3 consecutive days with an absolute neutrophil count greater than 0.5×10^9 /L (plus >20×10^9 /L platelets and hemoglobin >80 g/L, transfusion-free). The incidence of graft failure occurs in < 3-5% in autologous and allogeneic transplantation, but increases to 10% in haploidentical transplantation. The causes associated with the development of graft failure are: insufficient conditioning, donor cell abnormalities, host abnormalities, drugs, infections, immune rejection, or low CD34 (1). Engraftment time is approximately 15-20 days with peripheral blood progenitors, 20-25 from bone marrow and 23-35 days from umbilical cord. Engraftment failure is defined as a neutrophil count <0.5×10^9 /L, platelets <20×10^9 /L and hemoglobin <8 dg/L at 28, 35 and 42 days (peripheral blood, bone marrow, and cord blood respectively) after infusion.

The management of graft rejection should be initiated as soon as possible. The most recommended activities to follow are: stop all toxic drugs, treat infections, start G-CSF (granulocyte colony stimulating factors) administration, adjust immunosuppressive therapy and use thrombopoietin analogues. (1).

F. Graft syndrome:

It is due to the reconstitution of the immune system after HSCT. It manifests as a high and well-tolerated fever of non-infectious origin caused by the development of the first neutrophils in peripheral blood indicating that engraftment has occurred. The pathogenesis of this syndrome is due to endothelial damage produced by the massive release of proinflammatory cytokines, C-GSF, EPO and products of degranulation and oxidative metabolism of neutrophils. Prophylaxis of this syndrome consists of avoiding the use of G-CSF after transplantation in high-risk patients. Treatment consists of suspending G-CSF immediately; if fever persists more than 48 hours after starting antibiotics, treatment with corticosteroids must be initiated. (20).

3.3.Invasive fungal infection

Invasive fungal infection (IFI) is the most common fungal infection in patients with hematologic diseases and hematopoietic stem cell transplantation with high morbidity and mortality. The average mortality rate is over 50% in these patient groups. Therefore, a critical assessment of the individual risk of IFI per patient is key in order to select the best prophylactic and/or therapeutic approach to increase the survival of these patients. (21).

The most frequent etiological agent in these infections is Aspergillus fumigatus (Figure 1), a type of filamentous fungus, but we note a considerable increase in other species capable of causing this invasive disease belonging to the same genus Aspergillus and other different ones such as Fusarium, Scedosporium and mucorales fungi (21). (21). Invasive fungal infection caused by Aspergillus is called invasive aspergillosis (IA).

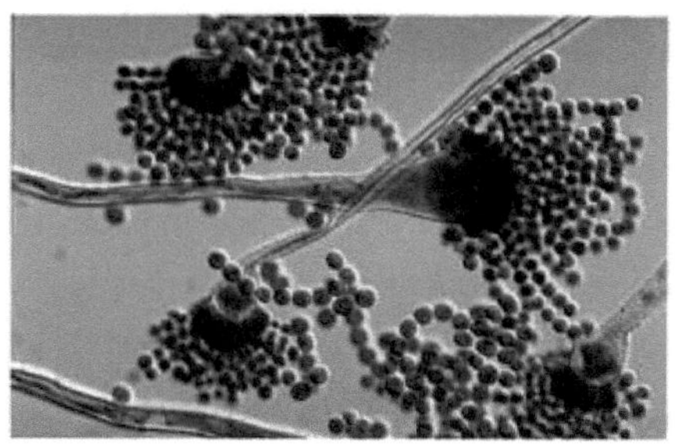

Figure 1. Image of *Aspergillus* under the microscope (22).

The most frequent risk periods include the pre-engraftment period, the post-engraftment period (between days +40 and +100) and the late post-transplant period (from day +100). During the pre-engraftment period when neutropenia and mucosal damage is most severe. In the post-engraftment period because patients are at higher risk for graft versus host disease and viral reactivations due to defects in T-cell immunity. During the late post-transplant period because of chronic GVHD, delayed recovery of the immune system and occasionally, because of secondary neutropenia (22).

Before the introduction of antifungal prophylaxis, the prevalence of Candida infections, a yeast-like fungus (Figure 2), in HSCT was 18-20% (22). (22). However, the use of prophylactic fluconazole in 1990 significantly reduced the incidence of systemic candidemia and has also decreased mortality secondary to systemic Candida infections. But this success of prophylaxis quickly became a generator of Candida resistance and made C. krusei and C.glabrata species the most predominant ones (23). In the last two decades, respiratory fungal infections caused by Aspergillus spp. have become the most prevalent. The mode of infection of yeasts is usually by venous or intestinal routes, unlike infections by other fungi which are acquired by inhalation of spores. In patients undergoing TMCH, the first lines of defense such as alveolar macrophages and neutrophils are usually non-functional. In addition, Aspergillus spores germinate and emit hyphae that invade blood vessels, causing venous occlusion and dissemination to other organs, resulting in fatal outcomes such as death in 60% of patients. (1).

In the context of HSCT, invasive aspergillosis can occur in two phases. Early IA is influenced by the underlying disease and age of the patient, the use of cord blood as a source of progenitors and cytomegalovirus (CMV) disease. In late post-transplant IA, the most important risk factor is extensive chronic graft-versus-host disease (GVHD), during which, along with profound immunodeficiency, there is a qualitative alteration of neutrophil function (24). There are more risk criteria for IFI listed in the following table:

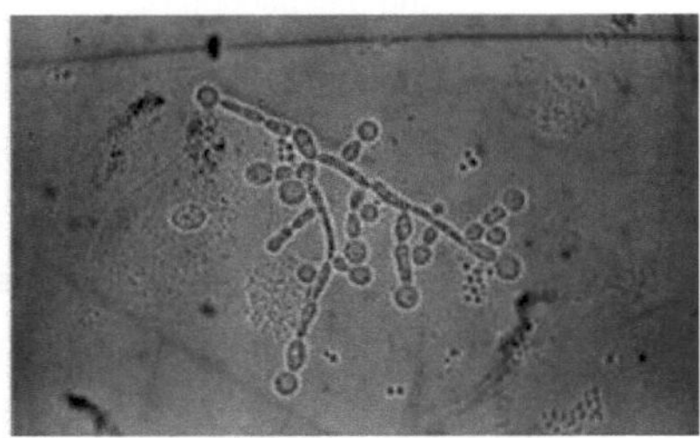

Figure 2. Image of *Candida* under the microscope (24).

Risk criteria for invasive fungal disease according to the consensus proposed by the European Organization for Research and Treatment of Cancer/Invasive Fungal Infections Cooperative Group and Infectious Diseases Mycoses Study Group (EORTC/MSG) (2020). (25):

Host criteria	Clinical criteria	Microbiological criteria
-Recent history of neutropenia (<0.5x10^9 neutrophils/L >10 days).	-Fungal disease of the lower respiratory tract (exclude alternative etiology). Presence on radiologic imaging of 1/3: dense, well-demarcated lesions with or without a halo sign, air crescent sign, or cavitated nodule.	-Direct tests: cytology, direct microscopy or direct culture of fungi or yeasts.
-Allogeneic transplant recipient.	Tracheobronchitis or tracheobronchial ulceration.	-Indirect tests: galactomannan and PCR in *Aspergillus*.
-Hematologic disease.	-Nasosinusal infection.	
-Prolonged use of corticosteroids (0.3 mg/kg/day of prednisone or equivalent > 3 weeks.	-Infection of the central nervous system.	
-Treatment with immunosuppressive agents such as cyclosporine, anti-TNF-α, certain monoclonal antibodies or nucleoside analogues during the last 90 days.	-Disseminated Candidiasis.	

Host criteria	**Clinical criteria**	**Microbiological criteria**
-Severe hereditary immunodeficiency (such as chronic granulomatous disease or severe combined immunodeficiency).		
Grade III or IV acute GVHD (intestinal, pulmonary or hepatic) refractory to first-line steroid therapy.		

3.4.Most common causative agents

Aspergillus

There are more than 250 species of *Aspergillus*, but the most common include *A. fumigatus* (57%), *A. flavus* (12%), *A. terreus* (12%), and *A. niger* (10%). (26). These are the opportunistic pathogenic fungi that most commonly affect immunocompromised patients (27). The genus *Aspergillus* typically affects the lungs, causing aspergillomas, hypersensitivity-related diseases such as allergic asthma, pneumonitis or allergic bronchopulmonary aspergillosis. Immunosuppressed patients are most at risk for the disseminated and invasive forms of aspergillosis (28). It can also affect organs such as the eyes and cause endophthalmitis to the central nervous system and cause brain abscesses and encephalopathy (29). *Aspergillus* species are mainly found in the external environment around us, in soils, vegetation and seeds, but can also be found indoors. Infection is acquired via inhalation of conidia into the lungs, causing activation of the innate and adaptive immune response. (26). Macrophages present in the airways contribute to phagocytosis and production of secondary mediators that recognize beta-D-glucan cell walls. In this way, neutrophils are recruited and cellular immunity is activated, causing the destruction of the organism. In other cases, the infection can spread through the blood and anchor itself in other organs such as the nervous or circulatory system (28).

Candida

Several *Candida* species are implicated in causing various diseases such as *C. Albincans, C. krusei, C. glabrata C. tropicalis, C. lusitaniae* and *C. parapsilosis in* both immunocompromised and immunocompetent patients. *Parapsilosis* in both immunocompromised and immunocompetent patients. *Candida* is a ubiquitous microorganism in the environment. The immune response to *Candida* depends on the location of the fungus. When it is found in the oropharynx, the local defense is the generation of proteins included in the saliva that hinder adhesion and growth. (30). In the case of disseminated infections, innate immunity plays a decisive role in killing *Candida*. Neutrophils and monocytes recognize the fungal surface and opsonize and kill the fungus by oxidative mechanisms. Endothelial cells secrete proinflammatory mediators that help resist vascular invasion. Humoral immunity also plays an important role in complement activation to recruit phagocytes to aid in the destruction of the organism. (28).

Pneumocystis

For decades, *Pneumocystis* was thought to be a protozoan, but it was eventually discovered to be a single-celled fungus. The species *Pneumocystis jirovecii* is responsible for causing pathology in humans. Patients with HSCT and other hematologic diseases are particularly susceptible to this infection. Symptoms of the disease include cough, fever, weight loss, and even respiratory failure. (28).

Mucormycosis

The vast majority of mucoralese fungi that infect humans are of the genera *Rhizopus, Mucor and Lichtheimia*. These species are usually found in decaying organic matter. Infection is acquired by airborne inhalation of spores or directly by inoculation through altered mucous membranes. As a result, in addition to localization in the respiratory tract, these species can cause disseminated disease, especially in immunocompromised patients, such as HCTs. (28). Survival depends on prompt diagnosis and treatment. Mortality was as high as 88% in the 1960s, whereas it is now around 15% (31). (31).

3.5.Diagnosis of fungal infections

Filamentous fungi:

The diagnosis of invasive filamentous fungal infections is still a challenge. Clinical manifestations in HSCT patients are nonspecific and difficult to distinguish from other non-fungal infections and non-infectious complications. Diagnosis is based on histopathological examination of infected tissues, thoracic CT imaging, and microbiological cultures (1). Although histopathology techniques are the gold-standard, many physicians refuse to perform invasive procedures in this type of patient because of possible complications or underlying coagulation problems; therefore, most infections are categorized as probable or possible and treatment is completely empirical. Microbiological cultures have the advantages of allowing identification of the causative agent, but they are time consuming and require expertise. In addition, blood cultures are usually negative for fungi, even in disseminated infections, and sputum cultures have moderate sensitivity and predictive value. (1).

The development of serological tests has been the major advance. Galactomannan is a molecule that is part of the fungal cell wall and is released during growth, which means that it can be detected by commercial enzyme immunoassay techniques. (32) (33). Previously, studies determined the positive test when the index was greater than or equal to 1.5. Currently the ECIL guidelines give the result as positive when the index is greater than or equal to 0.7 or repeated 0.5. This allows the detection of fungal infections before clinical-radiological manifestations appear. However, increasing sensitivity by lowering the cut-off points results in a loss of specificity. In addition, false positive and false negative results are quite frequent and cross-reactivity with other *non-Aspergillus* species, including *Fusarium spp, Penicillium spp, Acremonium spp, Alternaria spp, and Histoplasma capsulatum,* often occurs even though the technique is not capable of detecting mucorales.

The sensitivity and specificity of conventional radiology are very low for diagnosing or excluding fungal infections. Lung computed tomography is rapidly gaining popularity as a diagnostic technique. The appearance of pulmonary nodules with or without halo signs in the findings are suggestive of invasive fungal disease. The halo sign appears early in the course of the infection and later, these lesions become more nonspecific. (34).

Yeast:

Microbiological cultures are the gold-standard for the diagnosis of invasive *Candida* infections and candidemia, but they have low sensitivity, especially for chronic disseminated candidiasis. In addition, cultures take about five days to grow. Automated panels are being developed to diagnose candidemia in blood and identify the *Candida* species in less than five hours (35).

β-d-glucan is a component of the wall of many fungi such as *Candida spp, Fusarium spp*, and *Pneumocystis*. The tests used for diagnosis give results with good sensitivity, but low in specificity and positive predictive values due to the high false positive rate (32) (33).

Pneumocystis jirovecii:

Immunofluorescence assays are the most sensitive microscopic method. Real-time PCR in bronchoalveolar fluid can be used for the diagnosis of Pneumocystis. However, a positive result does not mean that the patient has the infection, as low fungal loads from colonized patients yield positive results (36).

3.6.Objectives

The main objective of this Master's thesis is to review invasive fungal infections in a special type of population, such as HSCT patients. As well as, to know the methods of prophylaxis and treatment, describing the most used antifungal drugs.

As secondary objectives, the aim is to provide information on hematologic transplant patients and the characteristics that predispose them to suffer these infections.

4. Material and Methods

Design: A review of documents from scientific societies, systematic reviews and scientific studies dedicated to hematopoietic transplants and the description of fungal infections as one of the most common complications in these patients was carried out.

Search strategy: A search was carried out in the Pubmed, Cochrane Library and Science Direct databases for documents and clinical practice guidelines published by different Spanish and international societies. The search was conducted in English. The following keywords and logical connectors were used for the search:

"HSCT AND fungal infections; Invasive fungal infections; Aspergillosis AND treatment; Candidiasis AND treatment."

We limited the search years to 10, although we also reviewed the original bibliographic references that appeared in the articles in order to select other studies that could potentially be included in this review.

Inclusion and exclusion criteria: Inclusion criteria were that the studies should be in English, incorporate recommendations on the management of fungal infections in patients undergoing hematopoietic stem cell transplantation, appropriate use of antifungals, and routine clinical practice guidelines.

The main exclusion criteria were: the articles did not include information on the use of antifungals in hematopoietic transplant patients and/or did not refer to prophylaxis and treatment guidelines. Articles published prior to 2012.

Data extraction: After the initial search, 1,113 studies were located, although 897 were excluded in the screening after applying "review, systematic review and 10-year" filters. With the following reviews, 149 studies that were not relevant to the objective of this review were discarded. Finally, 105 articles were selected, including 15 systematic reviews, 8 clinical practice guidelines and 82 original articles, which included recommendations from various professional societies.

To proceed to the final selection, we reviewed the abstracts and, if necessary, the conclusions of the articles in order to conclude whether or not the information they contained was related to the objective of our study and met the inclusion criteria.

In the following flowchart, the screening after the review is represented.

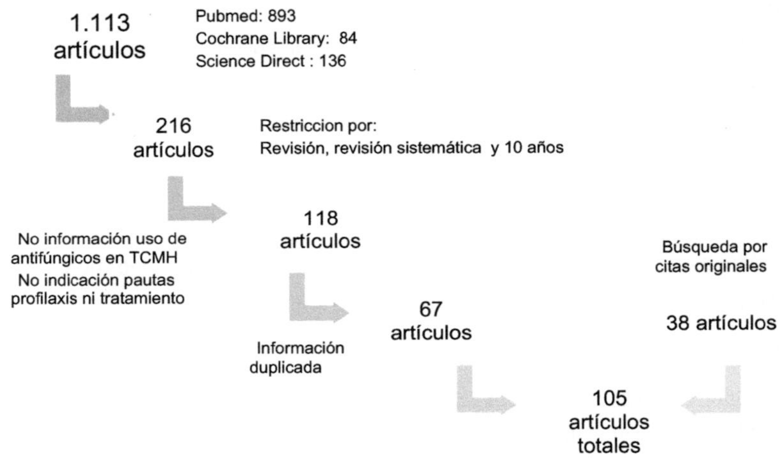

5. Results and discussion

As mentioned above, the infections suffered by the neutropenic patient are the most important and serious complications. In this section we will focus on the approach to fungal infections, from the prophylaxis indicated to prevent infections in these patients to the treatment once signs of disease appear.

5.1. Prophylaxis

Prophylactic measures are primarily aimed at preventing the acquisition of IA-causing agents from the air surrounding the patient and thus avoiding colonization of the bronchial tree. The use of HEPA filters in isolation rooms are very useful to avoid hospital acquisition of these pathogens (37) (38).

Currently, azole antifungals are the most widely used drugs for prophylaxis in populations at high risk for IA, such as patients with acute myeloid leukemia, myelodysplastic syndrome, patients with severe and persistent neutropenia, those with allogeneic transplantation (HSCT) during the neutropenia phase, and those with immunosuppression (39). (39)(40). The optimal duration of antifungal prophylaxis against filamentous fungi is not entirely clear. Thus, in patients who remain neutropenic it is logical to maintain it until complete recovery of neutropenia is achieved and in the case of patients with GVHD until the activity of the outbreak is controlled (41) (42).

Recommendations for antifungal prophylaxis are phase specific:

During the pre-graft neutropenia phase, fluconazole at a dose of 400 mg per day is the most recommended in sites with low incidence of filamentous fungus. In places with a higher incidence of filamentous fungal infections, other alternatives such as voriconazole should be adopted. Another alternative would also be micafungin. In places with a higher incidence of filamentous fungal infections, the addition of aerosolized liposomal amphotericin B to the treatment is recommended. Although there are no specific trial data on the use of posaconazole in prophylaxis, this drug is positioned as an alternative to the usual prophylaxis in neutropenic patients with acute myeloid leukemia and myelodysplastic syndrome (40). According to the meta-analysis conducted by

Wang et.al, with the review of 69 randomized clinical trials comparing 12 different antifungal treatments, they concluded that voriconazole is the most indicated antifungal for prophylaxis in patients with HSCT, while posaconazole is the best option for prophylaxis in patients with myeloid leukemia and myelodysplastic syndrome (43).

During the post-graft phase, with the high risk of infection that occurs during graft-versus-host complications, guidelines recommend the use of posaconazole for prophylaxis of these patients (40).

Pneumocystis jirovecii prophylaxis with trimethoprim and oral sulfamethoxazole 2 or 3 times a week is the guideline of choice. It should be given during the entire risk period, i.e., from engraftment to more than 6 months. Other drugs such as inhaled pentamidine, atovaquone or dapsone are second-line alternatives when trimethoprim and sulfamethoxazole are contraindicated or poorly tolerated. (33).

According to IDSA and ASCO guidelines, antifungal prophylaxis is recommended with an oral triazole or intravenous echinocandins in patients with profound and prolonged neutropenia, such as those affected by leukemia, myeloproliferative syndromes and HSCT (44). (44). In addition, prophylaxis is also recommended in patients with grade III and IV mucositis, in which the risk of candidiasis is quite high. In patients who are at low risk of profound and prolonged neutropenia, antifungal prophylaxis is not recommended.

Responsible physicians must be able to differentiate between the risk of invasive candidiasis and other invasive fungal infections. Fluconazole has activity against yeasts, but not against filamentous fungi. However, echinocandins and azole antifungals such as posaconazole, voriconazole and isavuconazole are the most active agents against filamentous fungi. (45).

When the risk of invasive aspergillosis is greater than 6%, the inclusion of a triazole active against filamentous fungi is recommended in those patients with HSCT, leukemia and myeloproliferative syndromes. The risk of invasive fungal infections is higher in patients with advanced stage allogeneic stem cell transplantation and in patients suffering from graft versus host disease, so the addition of an active antifungal therapy should be considered (37) (46) (47) (48).

5.2.Treatment of fungal infections

For a long time, profound and prolonged neutropenia, accompanied by fever for 5-7 days, and with broad-spectrum antibiotic coverage has been the trigger for initiating broad-spectrum antifungals, which is defined as empirical antifungal therapy (49). This practice has never been supported on a scientific basis and has significant drawbacks, including drug toxicity and increased treatment costs. Despite that, empiric therapy remains the standard of treatment in most centers. Considering that, ECIL guidelines recommend the use of caspofungin (70 mg as a loading dose and thereafter 50 mg daily) or liposomal amphotericin B at a rate of 3 mg/ kg (40).

Diagnosis-guided therapy, also called **anticipatory therapy**, is being implemented in many centers due to improvements in diagnostic techniques. The goal of this therapy is to initiate it in high-risk patients only when there are early markers of fungal infection, such as galactomannan testing, or positive PCR, or imaging evidence suggestive of lesioning (1).

Targeted therapy is used in patients with proven or probable fungal infection:

Voriconazole and isavuconazole are recommended as the first line of treatment for invasive aspergillosis, including cerebral aspergillosis (50). In a randomized clinical trial, voriconazole and isavuconazole demonstrated equal efficacy, but isavuconazole has a better safety profile than voriconazole and fewer drug-drug interactions (51). The combination of two antifungal agents with different mechanisms of action, such as the administration of a triazole together with an echinocandin is not recommended because they have not demonstrated superiority over triazole monotherapy (52). Liposomal amphotericin B at 3 mg/kg is the most recommended alternative once the azoles cannot be used due to problems of intolerance, interactions with other drugs, previous exposure to azole antifungals as prophylaxis and due to problems of resistance to azoles (53). The usual duration is 6 to 12 weeks, followed by secondary prophylaxis in patients maintaining immunosuppressive therapy. During the first week of treatment, pulmonary lesions may appear enlarged on imaging tests; this appears to be associated with the normal disease process and does not correlate with worse outcome (1).

Treatment of mucormycosis includes control of the patient's underlying conditions, surgical debridement and antifungal therapy. For the time being, liposomal amphotericin B formulations at doses of 5-10 mg/kg are the first line of treatment (50) (54). Once the infection is controlled, posaconazole and isavuconazole can be used orally for maintenance therapy.

Hyalohyphomycoses are a heterogeneous group of fungi that include *Fusarium*, *Scedosporium*, *Acremonium*, and *Scopulariopsis* species. Clinical manifestations range from colonization to localized infections to invasive and disseminated infections. The first line of treatment for these infections includes voriconazole and surgical debridement. Posaconazole can be used as salvage therapy. Voriconazole is also the recommended treatment against Scedosporium infections (55).

Echinocandins are considered the first line for the treatment of systemic candidiasis and candidemia, followed by targeted therapy once the *Candida* species and antifungal susceptibility are known (56). (56). Catheter removal is the most recommended action in the case of systemic infections. The duration of treatment should be 14 days after the first blood culture is negative. It should be noted that resistance to echinocandins is increasing, especially in the case of *C. glabrata* and in the recent discoveries of other species (57).

High doses of trimethoprim and sulfamethoxazole is the treatment of choice for patients with *Pneumocystis jirovecii* infection. The alternative is primaquine and clindamycin. The duration of treatment is about 3 weeks, followed by secondary prophylaxis. (58).

Table 7 summarizes the antifungals used as first-line agents in the treatment of invasive aspergillosis and mucormycosis in patients undergoing hematopoietic transplantation, according to the ECIL guidelines, and Table 8 provides clarifications on the degree of recommendation and evidence of the European recommendations.

Although antifungal efficacy ratios are high for most IFIs, it is safety issues that limit the use of traditional antifungals in clinical practice. The polyene amphotericin B, an effective gold standard in the treatment of most IFIs, has been associated with increased adverse effects and requires extensive patient monitoring. Echinocandins provide additional options in the treatment of *Candida* or *Aspergillus* and are only available intravenously.

The azole drugs, the cornerstone of antifungal therapy, are limited by different spectra, by safety or by aspects of the pharmaceutical formulation. Fluconazole has no activity against *Aspergillus*, voriconazole is not effective against mucoralese agents and has a very relevant adverse effect profile as discussed in the section on this drug. Posaconazole, although it has a better antifungal spectrum, does not present greater clinical evidence regarding its effectiveness, so it has no official indications for the treatment of infections caused by *Aspergillus* or mucorales.

ECIL guideline recommendations on first-line antifungal agents for invasive aspergillosis and mucormycosis in HSCT patients (40). (40).

	Grade of recommendation	**Posology**
Invasive aspergillosis		
Voriconazole	AI	6 mg/kg every 12 hours on the first day, followed by 4 mg/kg every 12 hours.
Isavuconazole	AI	200 mg every 8 hours for 2 days, and continue with 200 mg daily.
Liposomal Amphotericin B	BI	3 mg/ kg / day

Amphotericin B lipid complex	BII	5 mg/ kg / day
Amphotericin B colloidal dispersion	CI	
Caspofungin	CII	
Itraconazole	CIII	
Anidulafungin + voriconazole combination	AI	
Invasive *mucormycosis*		
Amphotericin B deoxycholate	CII	
Liposomal Amphotericin B	BII	5 mg/kg / day
Amphotericin B lipid complex	BII	
Amphotericin B colloidal dispersion	CII	
Posaconazole	CIII	

Table 8. Clarification of the grade of recommendation and quality of evidence of the ECIL guideline. (40).

Grade of recommendation and quality of evidence ECIL	
Grade of recommendation	
A	Good evidence to recommend its use
B	Moderate evidence to support the recommendation
C	Low evidence to support the recommendation
Quality of evidence	
I	Evidence of ≥ 1 adequate randomized, controlled trial.
II	Evidence from ≥ 1 well-designed clinical trial, without randomization; from analytical cohort or case-controlled studies; from multiple time series; or from dramatic results from uncontrolled experiments
III	Evidence of opinions from respected authorities based on clinical experience, descriptive studies or expert committee reports.

That is why the Spanish Society of Infectious Diseases and Microbiology (SEIMC) positions voriconazole and isavuconazole as first-line agents for the treatment of IA in hematological patients. Amphotericin B is considered an alternative treatment for those patients who cannot tolerate azole or allergic derivatives, who have suffered hepatic adverse effects, under therapeutic effect or who are under treatment with drugs that interact with them. The use of echinocandins (caspofungin, micafungin or anidulafungin) is only recommended as rescue combination therapy or in those cases that do not allow the use of azoles or amphotericin B (39).

Thus, second-line treatment varies according to the initial first-line treatment given to the patient. Thus, monotherapy with an antifungal of a different class is used (for example, use of liposomal amphotericin B after treatment with an azole or vice versa) or, if a combination treatment is decided upon, an echinocandin is added to the first-line treatment with azoles or liposomal amphotericin B (39).

5.3.Description of most commonly used drugs

This section describes the most commonly used antifungal drugs for prophylaxis and treatment of fungal infections occurring in HSCT patients.

The following image (Figure 3) visually summarizes the antifungal drugs and their target of action, which will be developed below (59).

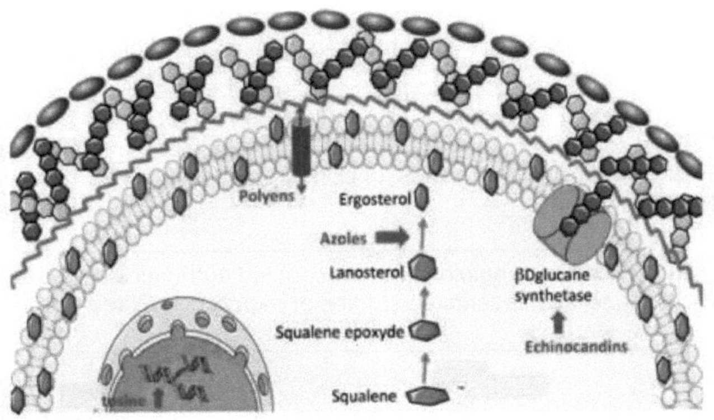

Figure 3. Pharmacological targets of antifungals (59)

5.3.1.Azole antifungals

Azole antifungals can be classified into imidazoles (ketoconazole) and triazoles (fluconazole, itraconazole, voriconazole, posaconazole, and isavuconazole) according to their chemical structure. The triazoles are the most widely used antifungals for both prophylaxis and treatment, as discussed in previous sections, since they have activity against most pathogenic fungi without the serious nephrotoxic effects observed with amphotericin B. The new azoles have become the standard of care for many fungal infections.

The fluorinated triazole antifungals (fluconazole, voriconazole, isavuconazole and posaconazole) are drugs with a triazole chemical structure, with three nitrogen atoms in their structure. To achieve better in vitro activity, the inclusion of fluorine atoms in the structure was tested. In this way, greater inhibitory activity was achieved and the spectrum of activity against fungal species that were inert to the initial compound was increased. (60).

The mechanism of action consists in the inhibition of 14-alpha-lanosterol demethylation mediated by the cytochrome P450-dependent enzyme lanosterol 14-alpha-demethylase, which is an essential step in fungal cell membrane biosynthesis: ergosterol. The accumulation of 14-alpha-methylsterols correlates with an accumulation of methylated sterol precursors and the consequent loss of ergosterol in the fungal cell membrane, leading to a weakening of the structure and function of the fungal cell membrane (61).

The mechanisms of azole resistance that have been described are: a) activation of alternative metabolic pathways, b) modifications of the ERG11 gene, which encodes 14-lanosterol demethylase, producing enzymes with lower affinity, c) overexpression of the previous gene, and d) induction of active expulsion systems. Most of these mechanisms are described for yeasts, but some also appear in the case of filamentous fungi (60).

All azole antifungals interact to a greater or lesser extent with cytochromes and other enzymes. Although it will be developed specifically in the section on each azole, the interactions of these antifungals with the enzymes responsible for metabolism are summarized in Table 9 below (59).

Table 9. Interactions of azole antifungals with enzymes involved in phase 1 and 2 metabolism and transporter proteins (59).

	Voriconazole	Isavuconazole	Posaconazole	Fluconazole
Phase 1 enzymes				

CYP 3A4/5	I S	I S	I	I S
CYP 2B6	I	I	-	-
CYP 2C9	I S	-	-	I S
CYP2C19	I S	-	-	I S
Phase 2 enzymes				
UGT	-	I	S	I
Transporter proteins				
P-glycoprotein	-	I	I S	S
BCRP	-	I	I	-
OCT2	-	I	-	-

Abbreviations: CYP, cytochromes; UGT, uridine diphosphate glucuronosyltransferase; BCRP, breast cancer resistance protein; OCT2, organic cation transporter type 2; I, metabolic inhibitor; S, enzyme substrate.

Voriconazole

Triazole derivative antifungal (Figure 4) with indications approved by the Spanish Agency of Medicines and Health Products (AEMPS) for the treatment of IA, candidemia in non-neutropenic patients, severe invasive *Candida* infections (including *C. krusei)* resistant to fluconazole, severe fungal infections by *Scedosporium spp.* and *Fusarium spp,* and also as prophylaxis of IFI in high-risk

HSCT recipients. (61) (62). Since was introduced in therapeutics in 2002, it has

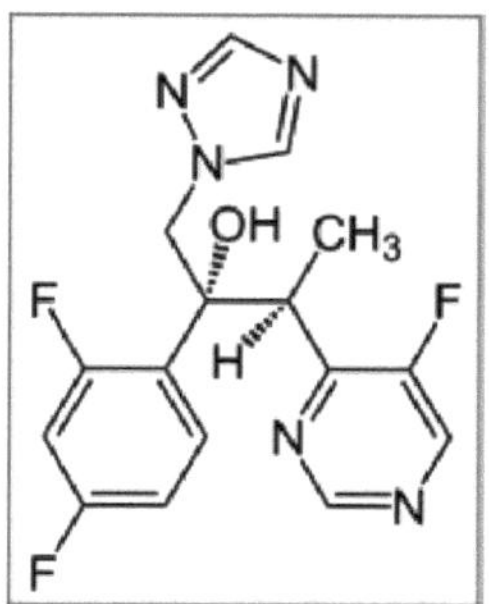

Figure 4. Chemical structure of voriconazole (64)

been positioned as the treatment of choice for invasive aspergillosis (63).

It is recommended to administer a loading dose on the first day to reach steady state. Intravenously, the loading dose is 6 mg/kg/12 hours and the maintenance dose is 4 mg/kg/12 hours. Given the good oral bioavailability (96%), administration by this route is recommended whenever possible. The loading dose used orally is 400 mg every 12 hours in adults weighing more than 40 kg and children over 15 years of age. The maintenance dose is 200 mg every 12 hours. For children under 15 years of age or adults weighing less than 40 kg, the loading dose is 200 mg every 12 hours and the maintenance dose is 100 mg per 12 hours. (61).

Metabolism of voriconazole is hepatic and primarily by cytochrome P450 isoenzyme CYP2C19, and in the minority by CYP3A4 and CYP2C9. CYP2C19 genetic polymorphisms result in phenotypes of fast and slow metabolizers, causing approximately 30-50 % variation in plasma concentrations. It is for this reason that many authors advocate the need to genotype CYP2C19 as part of the monitoring of voriconazole concentrations in order to avoid adverse reactions (64) (65).

Given its mechanism of action and metabolism, there are many interactions because it is a potent inhibitor of the cytochrome isoenzymes (cytochrome P450,

CYP2C19, CYP2C9 and CYP3A4), which causes an increase in the plasma concentrations of the drugs metabolized through them. The following table summarizes the most relevant interactions included in the data sheet:

Table 10. Most relevant pharmacological interactions.

Drug	Mechanism	Result	Recommendation
Rifampicin	Enzyme induction	↓[Voriconazole].	Contraindicated
Carbamazepine	Enzyme induction	↓[Voriconazole].	Contraindicated
Barbiturates	Enzyme induction	↓[Voriconazole].	Contraindicated
Astemizole, cisapride, pimozide, quinidine and terfenadine	CYP3A4 Substrates	They can produce QTc interval prolongation and torsades de pointes.	Contraindicated
Efavirenz	CYP450 Inducer; CYP3A4 Inhibitor and Substrate		Contraindicated
Ergot alkaloids (ergotamine and	CYP3A4 substrates	Plasma concentrations of alkaloids are increased and	Contraindicated

dihydroergotamine)		ergotism may occur.	
Ritonavir	Potent CYP450 inducer; CYP3A4 inhibitor and substrate	↓[Voriconazole].	Contraindicated
St. John's wort	CYP450 Inducer; P-gp inducer	↓[Voriconazole].	Contraindicated
Cyclosporine	CYP3A4 Substrate	↑ [Cyclosporine].	Halve the dose of cyclosporine and monitor levels.
Tacrolimus	CYP3A4 substrate.	↑ [Tacrolimus].	Reduce tacrolimus dose to one-third and monitor.

One of the most relevant interactions in hematologic patients is with immunosuppressants. A pharmacokinetic study in eleven HSCT patients with stable plasma levels of tacrolimus started on voriconazole showed a 116% increase in the concentration/dose ratio of tacrolimus after 7-10 days of treatment (66).

The most frequent adverse reactions are hepatotoxicity (defined as an increase in transaminases twice the limit of normal) which occurs in 20% of patients treated with voriconazole, but which does not require discontinuation of treatment (67). The most important risk factors for possible hepatotoxicity are chronic hepatic pathology and high blood drug levels (63). The technical data sheet recommends monitoring transaminase levels at the beginning and during treatment with voriconazole. Visual disturbances appear in 19 to 30% of patients (68). These alterations appear as problems in differentiating colors, blurred vision, bright spots and photophobia, which are reversible and disappear when treatment ceases. (68). Fever (5.7%), nausea (5.4%) and pruritus (5.3%) are also common. Photosensitivity may appear in 1-2% of patients treated with long therapies and may be a predisposing factor for malignant skin pathologies. This is due to the inhibitory action of voriconazole on the cytochrome enzymes CYP3A4 and CYP2C9, which are responsible for retinol metabolism, thus resulting in the accumulation of the toxic metabolite tretinoin (69). Photosensitivity reactions include erythema, cheilitis, lentigines, desquamation, hyperpigmentation and cutaneous pseudoporphyria (characterized by blistering, fragility and scarring). Photosensitivity may persist for months even after therapy has been terminated (69).

Other less common but no less important adverse reactions are: malignant skin pathologies, cardiac arrhythmias, periostitis, neurological effects, alopecia and nail changes. (63). The use of voriconazole in prolonged therapies over time may increase the risk of producing skin cancer and the mechanisms proposed to explain this are the potentiation of the action of UV rays, DNA damage and reduction of DNA repair mechanisms (70). However, given the small number of reported cases, a firm conclusion cannot be drawn (63). Cardiac arrhythmias are other less common adverse reactions that occur due to inhibition of fast potassium channels in cardiac tissue, causing an increase in the Q-T interval. Pharmacokinetic monitoring of voriconazole levels seems to be unable to prevent cardiac accidents since it appears to be due to the synergistic effect with other arrhythmogenic drugs (71). One of the most painful complications of voriconazole treatment is periostitis, because the drug contains 15 times the usual daily amount of fluoride. Studies analyzed plasma fluoride levels and found that their figures were above the usual levels. In addition, half of them developed periostitis (72). The neurological effects appear to be dependent on the blood concentration of the drug (73). Auditory and visual hallucinations are described. In addition, cases of peripheral neuropathies have also been described and the symptoms are usually paresthesias in the hands and feet or even weakness in the lower limbs (74).

Pharmacokinetic monitoring of voriconazole is recommended to reduce the occurrence of adverse effects due to the presence of supratherapeutic blood concentrations and to improve effectiveness in patients with subtherapeutic levels. (75). Trough concentration determination is used to adjust antifungal doses (between 1 and 5 µg/mL). For the levels obtained to be significant, the concentrations must have been obtained at steady state, which is reached 48 hours after treatment provided that a loading dose has been administered and 6 days without a loading dose. (76).

Despite interactions and adverse effects, the efficacy of voriconazole has been proven in numerous comparative studies with other antifungals. Some examples are discussed below. In the study by Herbrecht (77) study compared the efficacy of voriconazole versus amphotericin B in the treatment of IA in neutropenic and HSCT patients. It was shown to be superior in efficacy (55% vs. 38%) and improved survival at 12 weeks after transplantation (71% vs. 58%) with fewer adverse events. In other studies, the activity of lipid amphotericin B was compared against voriconazole, concluding in lower in vitro activity against *Aspergillus* *nidulans* species, *lentulus* and terreus (62) (63).

Isavuconazole

Iavuconazonium sulfate, a prodrug of isavuconazole (Figure 5 (78)), is available as an oral and intravenous formulation, with the great advantage that since it is highly water soluble, its intravenous formulation does not require the use of cyclodextrins (required in the intravenous formulations of other azole antifungals such as voriconazole, itraconazole and posaconazole), thus eliminating the nephrotoxicity associated with this vehicle. Both orally and intravenously, 372 mg of isavuconazonium sulfate is rapidly metabolized (prodrug and inactive metabolite indectable within 30 minutes of intravenous infusion) by the body's esterases into 200 mg of the active drug, isavuconazole; just as 186 mg of the prodrug gives rise to 100 mg of isavuconazole (79). Unlike other azoles, the pharmacokinetics of isavuconazole are not affected by the use of proton pump inhibitors or other drugs that alter gastric pH such as H2-receptor antagonists.

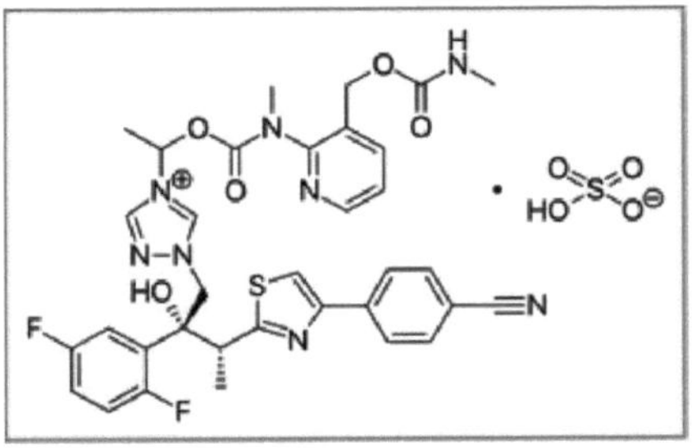

Figure 5. Chemical structure of isavuconazole (81)

It is a drug with high oral bioavailability (98%), which is not affected by food intake, with linear, dose-dependent pharmacokinetics and low interindividual variability. In healthy individuals and in a group of patients with acute myeloid leukemia and neutropenia, maximum concentrations (Cmax) in the steady state were found to be 2.5 ±1.0 μg/mL (80). However, pharmacokinetic monitoring is not routinely recommended since there is no clear dose-response relationship and interindividual variability of plasma levels is low (81).

The toxicity profile is similar to that of other triazoles with gastrointestinal alterations but apparently, although with limited evidence, less incidence of photosensitivity, skin alterations, as well as hepatobiliary and visual alterations compared to voriconazole. Phase I and II studies do not demonstrate serious side effects, the most frequent being: abdominal pain, moderate conjunctivitis, diarrhea, flu-like syndrome, and moderate dizziness and nausea. (82). However, serious cutaneous adverse reactions, such as Stevens-Johnson syndrome, have been reported. Unlike the other azoles, it decreases QT.

It is indicated for the treatment of invasive aspergillosis and mucormycosis in patients for whom amphotericin B is not appropriate.

Approval for use in invasive aspergillosis is based on the results of a randomized, double-blind, non-inferiority study comparing isavuconazole and voriconazole for the treatment of invasive aspergillosis and other fungal invasive infections (51). In which a total of 516 adult patients with proven, possible or probable invasive fungal infection defined by EORTC/MSG criteria were randomized 1:1 to receive either isavuconazole or voriconazole. The results of the SECURE clinical trial determine the non-inferiority of isavuconazole versus voriconazole with the primary endpoint being all-cause mortality at 42 days (18.6% vs. 20.2%). In addition, this trial shows a better safety profile for isavuconazole versus voriconazole [adverse events reported in isavuconazole and voriconazole, 42% versus 60%, respectively, (p<0.001)] and a lower incidence of drug-drug interactions in isavuconazole.

The efficacy of isavuconazole in the treatment of mucormycosis has only been proven through an uncontrolled open-label clinical trial with 37 patients (83). Patients received isavuconazole at a dosage similar to that of the SECURE study until resolution of the condition, therapeutic failure, or completion of 180 days of treatment; patients were compared with a control group that had received amphotericin B. The main variable was the response to treatment (complete or complete). The primary endpoint was response to treatment (complete or partial). Mortality at day 42 from the start of treatment was similar to that reported in the registry for patients treated with amphotericin B: 33% (isavuconazole) vs. 39% (amphotericin B). (83).

Its antifungal spectrum similar to that of voriconazole, including the main species of *Aspergillus ssp*, mucorales and fluconazole-resistant *Candida krusei* species (84).

Safety data for isavuconazole, as discussed, are limited due to its short experience in clinical use; in the SECURE study, no significant differences were observed between patients who had adverse reactions with voriconazole (98%) or isavuconazole (96%). However, patients treated with isavuconazole had a significantly lower proportion of ocular, hepatobiliary, and cutaneous toxicity (51).

The proportion of patients with drug-attributable adverse effects was also lower in the group receiving isavuconazole versus that receiving voriconazole, just as the proportion of patients who had to discontinue treatment due to drug-attributable toxicity was lower in the isavuconazole group compared to the voriconazole group (14% vs. 23%) (51).

Drug interactions with cytochrome-metabolized drugs are expected, especially with CYP3A4 substrates and inducers, since in vitro/in vivo studies indicate that both CYP3A4 and CYP3A5 and subsequent uridine diphosphate glucuronosyltransferase (UGT) substrates are involved in the metabolism of isavuconazole. Drugs that induce these enzymes increase the levels of the antifungal drug: ketoconazole, high doses of ritonavir, as well as potent inducers. In addition, isavuconazole is a moderate CYP3A4/5 inhibitor so that co-administration with other drugs metabolized by this pathway will cause an increase in the plasma concentrations of these drugs with the clinical repercussions that this entails, both in efficacy and toxicity. The latter situation is the most common and relevant in clinical practice.

The interactions listed in the data sheet are summarized in the following table (
table 11) (85):

Table 11. Most relevant pharmacological interactions of isavuconazole.

Drug	Mechanism	Result	Recommendation
Carbamazepine, phenobarbital and phenytoin	Potent CYP3A4 enzyme induction	↓[Isavuconazole].	Contraindicated
Rifampicin	Potent CYP3A4 enzyme induction	↓[Isavuconazole].	Contraindicated

St. John's wort	Potent CYP3A4 enzyme induction	↓[Isavuconazole].	Contraindicated
Cyclosporine, tacrolimus	CYP3A4 Substrates	↑[Cyclosporine]. ↑[Tacrolimus].	Control plasma levels
Cyclophosphamide	CYP2B6 Substrate	↓[Cyclophosphamide].	Monitor lack of efficacy, and if necessary increase the dose.
Ritonavir	Powerful inductor CYP3A4/5	↓[Isavuconazole].	contraindicated
Digoxin	P-gp substrate	↑[Digoxin].	Serum digoxin concentrations should be monitored.

It should be noted that it can increase plasma concentrations of atorvastatin, the immunosuppressants widely used in oncohematology (cyclosporine, sirolimus, tacrolimus and mycophenolate mofetil) in which doses should be closely monitored, and it also increases midazolam concentrations. In addition, since it is a moderate P-glycoprotein inhibitor, when used concomitantly with digoxin, plasma levels of digoxin may increase, and should therefore be closely monitored. (86).

The off-label use of antifungal prophylaxis in clinical practice has increased, especially in immunocompromised patients or those with oncohematological diseases when other azoles are contraindicated, and the literature or evidence available for this indication is quite limited. However, after searching in different databases, no systematic reviews, meta-analyses or randomized trials giving evidence for the use of isavuconazole as prophylaxis were found. Most of the published studies are case reviews or retrospective cohort studies with important limitations.

The study carried out by Fontana et al. shows important limitations as it is a retrospective and single-center study (N=145 patients) showing a higher incidence of IFI in patients treated with isavuconazole (8.1% of patients on prophylactic treatment develop IFI) (87). (87). Stern et al. developed a single-arm prospective open-label cohort study evaluating the use of isavuconazole for antifungal prophylaxis after HSCT. The data obtained support the usefulness of isavuconazole but reflect important limitations (88). Another retrospective cohort study conducted by Bowen et al. evaluates the economic impact showing a reduction in the cost of prophylactic treatment compared to posaconazole and with clinical results similar to those obtained by Fontana. IFI developed in 8.2% of the patients in the cohort, compared to 2.0% and 2.4% observed in clinical trials of posaconazole prophylaxis (89).

Only one clinical trial has evaluated the pharmacokinetics, safety and tolerability of isavuconazole for the prevention of fungal infections in patients with severe and prolonged neutropenia. An open-label multicenter phase 2 clinical trial (n=24), the investigators evaluated the safety and efficacy of isavuconazole prophylaxis in patients with LAM who developed febrile neutropenia post chemotherapy. The results of this analysis support the safety and tolerability of isavuconazole administered at 200 mg and 400 mg once daily as prophylaxis in immunosuppressed patients at high risk for fungal infections, with no cases of proven or probable IFI found during isavuconazole treatment (80).

Finally, isavuconazole may be an alternative in prophylaxis in immunocompromised patients or those at high risk of IFI, showing similar effectiveness and good adverse effect profile; however, these results support the need for further studies to determine the role of isavuconazole as prophylaxis in this population group, as well as the need for non-inferiority randomized clinical trials to provide evidence for its use.

Posaconazole

Posaconazole is a second-generation, broad-spectrum triazole (Figure 6) analog of itraconazole (90). (90). In Spain, the indications for which it is authorized are for: invasive aspergillosis in patients with disease resistant to amphotericin B or itraconazole, fusariosis in patients with disease resistant to amphotericin B, or due to intolerance to amphotericin B; chromoblastomycosis and mycetoma in patients with disease resistant to itraconazole, or in patients who are intolerant to itraconazole, coccidioidomycosis in patients with disease resistant to amphotericin B, itraconazole or fluconazole, or in patients who are intolerant to these drugs (91). It is also licensed for use in the prophylaxis of invasive fungal infections in patients receiving chemotherapy for acute myelogenous leukemia (AML) or myelodysplastic syndromes (MDS), and in hematopoietic stem cell transplant (HSCT) recipients who are receiving high doses of immunosuppressive therapy for graft-versus-host disease (GVHD), and who are at high risk for developing invasive fungal infections (91).

The recommended dose is 300 mg of posaconazole every 12 hours on the first day, and continue with 300 mg once daily. If used as prophylaxis, it should be started several days before the expected date of neutropenia and continued for 7 days after the neutrophil count exceeds 500 cells/ mm^3 . (91). In patients with renal insufficiency, accumulation of the intravenous vehicle sulfobutyl ether beta-cyclodextrin may occur. In such cases the administration of oral formulations is recommended. Administered orally, posaconazole is excreted mainly unchanged in feces (77%), making it a good alternative in patients with renal insufficiency, since it allows its administration without adjustment (92).

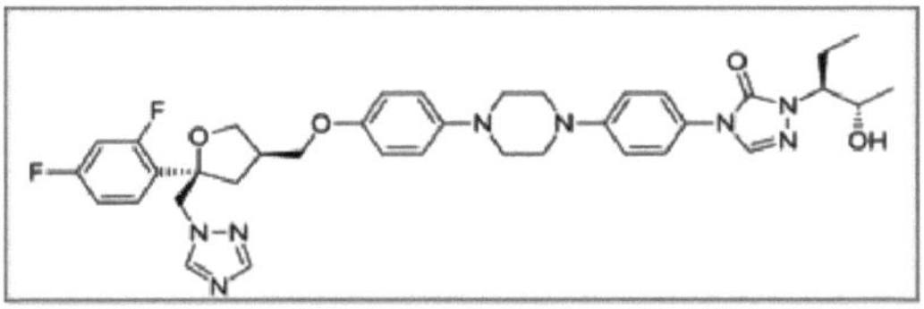

Figure 6. Chemical structure of posaconazole (93)

The long side chain of posaconazole allows for increased hydrophobic binding to CYP51, which results in achieving activity against fluconazole- and voriconazole-resistant species (93). Posaconazole has demonstrated excellent antifungal activity against *Candida* and *Aspergillus*, which are the main IFI-producing agents. Compared with other triazoles, posaconazole offers additional coverage against mucorals (94).

Recent meta-analyses position posaconazole as a good and effective therapeutic option for reducing the overall incidence of invasive fungal infections (95). Once comparative subgroup analyses were performed, it was concluded that fluconazole was superior to fluconazole in reducing the risk of IFI, thus positioning fluconazole as an improved alternative for the prevention of yeast infections instead of using it against filamentous fungi. However, with the use of fluconazole, some *Candida* species have developed resistance, leading to a reduction in the use of fluconazole and an increase in invasive aspergillosis in patients with HSCT (96).

There are few comparative efficacy and safety trials between posaconazole, voriconazole and isavuconazole.

Posaconazole is metabolized by glucuronidation with UDP (phase 2 enzymes) and is a substrate for p-glycoprotein (P-gp) efflux in vitro. Therefore, inhibitors and inducers of these clearance pathways may respectively increase or decrease plasma concentrations of posaconazole. Posaconazole is a CYP3A4 inhibitor. The most significant interactions are listed in Table 12.

The most common adverse effects of posaconazole are nausea, vomiting, diarrhea, headache and alterations in liver function. Comparison in terms of safety with other antifungal agents concluded that there were no significant differences. However, posaconazole should be used with caution in patients with comorbidities due to possible drug-drug interactions. (90).

Table 12. Most relevant interactions included in the data sheet.

Drug	**Mechanism**	**Result**	**Recommendatio n**

Phenytoin	Potent CYP3A4 enzyme induction	↓[Posaconazole].	Contraindicated
Rifabutin, rifampicin	Potent CYP3A4 enzyme induction	↓[Posaconazole].	Contraindicated
Fosamprenavir	CYP3A4 enzyme induction	↓[Posaconazole].	Monitor lack of efficiency
Efavirenz	Potent CYP3A4 enzyme induction	↓[Posaconazole].	Contraindicated
Cyclosporine, tacrolimus	CYP3A4 Substrates	↑[Cyclosporine]. ↑[Tacrolimus].	Reduce doses of immunosuppressants
Midazolam	CYP2B6 Substrate	↑[Midazolam].	Benzodiazepine dose adjustment
Sirolimus	CYP3A4 Substrates	↓[Isavuconazole].	Contraindicated
Digoxin	P-gp substrate	↑[Digoxin].	Serum digoxin concentrations should be monitored.

Fluconazole

Fluconazole is a triazole antifungal drug (Figure 7). (97)) whose administration is indicated in Spain for the treatment of cryptococcal meningitis, coccidioidomycosis, invasive candidiasis, mucosal candidiasis including oropharyngeal and esophageal candidiasis, candiduria and chronic mucocutaneous candidiasis and chronic atrophic oral candidiasis. In addition, it is also licensed for the prophylaxis of relapses of cryptococcal meningitis in patients at high risk of relapse, relapses of oropharyngeal and esophageal candidiasis in AIDS-infected patients who are at high risk of relapse, prophylaxis of Candida infections in patients with prolonged neutropenia (such as patients with hematologic malignancies receiving chemotherapy or patients receiving HSCT) (98).

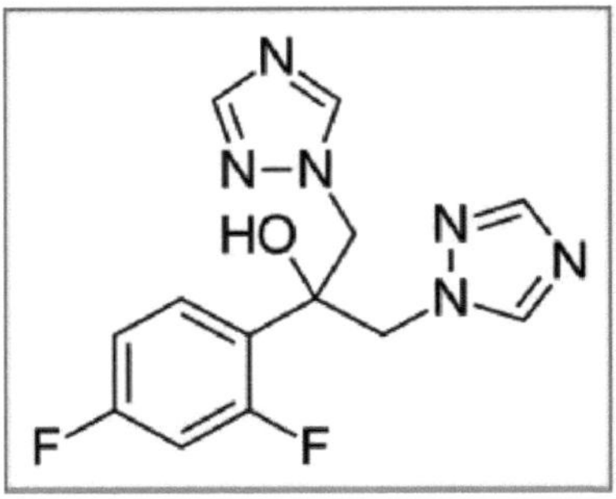

Figure 7. Chemical structure of fluconazole (97)

Fluconazole is a potent inhibitor of CYP2C9 and a moderate inhibitor of CYP3A4 and CYP2C19 isoenzymes. Table 13 lists the drugs whose interactions are the most relevant with fluconazole.

The most frequent adverse reactions are headache, nausea, vomiting, diarrhea, increased liver enzymes and skin rash.

Table 13. Table of the most relevant interactions included in the data sheet (98).

Drug	Mechanism	Result	Recommendation
Cisapride, terfenadine, astemizole, pimozide, quinidine, and erythromycin	CYP2C9 Substrates	↑[Pharmaceuticals]	Coadministration contraindicated
Amiodarone	CYP2C9 Substrates	↑[Amiodarone].	Use with caution
Phenytoin	Enzyme inhibition	↑[Phenytoin]	Monitor phenytoin levels
Rifabutin, rifampicin	Enzyme inhibition	↑[rifabutin and rifampicin].	Monitor for signs of toxicity
Oral anticoagulants	CYP2C9 Enzyme Inhibition	↑[Warfarin]	Anticoagulant dose adjustment
Cyclosporine, tacrolimus, sirolimus	CYP3A4 Substrates	↑[Cyclosporine]. ↑[Tacrolimus]. ↑[Sirolimus].	Reduce doses of immunosuppressants
Midazolam	CYP2B6 Substrate	↑[Midazolam].	Benzodiazepine dose adjustment

5.3.2.Echinocandins

There are three FDA-approved echinocandins: micafungin, anidulafungin and caspofungin (Figures 8, 9 and 10). (99) (100) (101)). Echinocandins are cyclic lipopeptides that represent the third group of antifungals available for the treatment of systemic fungal infections. Due to the increasing incidence of *Candida* species with resistance to fluconazole, echinocandins are playing a pivotal role in the treatment of this pathology (102).

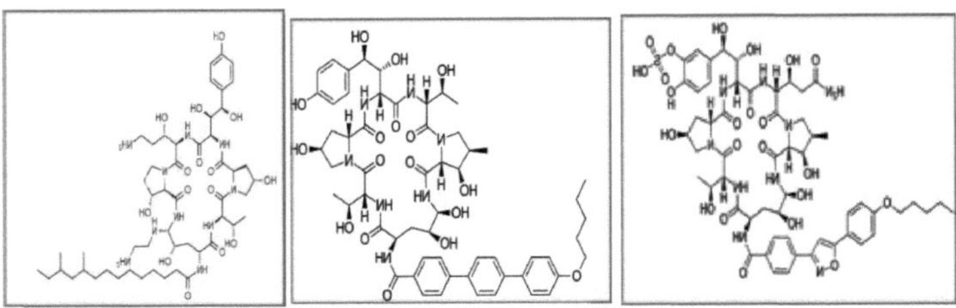

Figure 10. Chemical structure of caspofungin (101).

Figure 9. Chemical structure of anidulafungin (100)

Figure 8. Chemical structure micafungin (99)

The mechanism of action of echinocandins is the non-competitive inhibition of UDP-glucose β-(1,3)-D-glucan-β-(3)-D-glucosyltransferase (commonly referred to as 1,3-β-D glucan synthase), an enzyme required for the synthesis of 1,3-β-D glucan, an essential component of the fungal cell wall. For certain *Candida* species, inhibition of glucan synthase destabilizes the integrity of the cell wall, leaving it less rigid and unable to withstand changes in osmotic pressure, concluding in cell lysis (103).

The three echinocandins mentioned above show activity against *Candida* species: *C. albicans*, *C. glabrata*, *C. tropicalis*, *C. dubliniensis*, and *C. krusei*, which are resistant to amphotericin and fluconazole (103). For filamentous fungal species, such as those belonging to the *Aspergillus* species, 1,3-β-D glucan synthase is found mainly in the apical tips of the hyphae and has been determined to have fungistatic activity in vitro and in vivo (104).

Echinocandins are indicated for the treatment of oropharyngeal and esophageal candidiasis. Table 14 shows all the indications listed in the technical data sheet for each echinocandin. Although therapeutic guidelines recommend the administration of fluconazole, echinocandins are a good, effective and well-tolerated alternative. Moreover, they are considered an alternative for candidiasis refractory to first-line treatment. Due to cost and post-treatment relapse rates, echinocandins are not considered first-line treatment unless the causative agent is azole-resistant, intolerant, or has drug interactions (102).

Table 14. Summary of indications approved in the technical data sheet by the AEMPS for echinocandins.

Drug	**Approved indications in the data sheet**
Caspofungin	-Invasive candidiasis. -Invasive aspergillosis in adult or pediatric patients who are refractory or intolerant to amphotericin B, lipid formulations of amphotericin B and/or itraconazole. -Empirical treatment of fungal infections (such as *Candida* or *Aspergillus*) in adult or pediatric neutropenic patients with fever.
Micafungin	-Invasive candidiasis. -Esophageal candidiasis in patients in whom intravenous therapy is adequate. -Prophylaxis of *Candida* infection in patients undergoing allogeneic hematopoietic stem cell transplantation or in patients who are expected to have neutropenia for 10 or more days.
Anidulafungin	-Invasive candidiasis.

The mechanisms of resistance to echinocandins have been attributed to mutations in genes encoding for 1,3-β-D glucan synthase, specifically FKS1 and FKS2. Mutations in these genes result in alterations in the formation of the catalytic subunit of the enzyme complex, which is the main target of these drugs. These types of mutations are believed to result in cross-resistance for all agents in this group. Other proposed mechanisms of resistance include the presence of ejector pumps in the cell wall and an overexpression of transporter proteins (105) (106).

Due to their high molecular weight, none of them are absorbed when administered orally, so the presentations are intravenous. They have high protein binding. One of the main advantages is that none is significantly metabolized by cytochrome P450, nor is it a substrate of P-glycoprotein P (102). For this reason, there are no relevant drug-drug interactions. Caspofungin is the most CYP450-dependent echinocandin, whereas anidulafungin is the least. Drugs such as rifampicin, nevirapine, efavirenz, carbamazepine, dexamethasone and phenytoin induce the metabolism of caspofungin. The following table summarizes the most important interactions listed in the data sheet.

Table 15. Most relevant interactions of the echinocandins (caspofungin) included in the data sheet (107).

Drug	Mechanism	Result	Recommendation
Cyclosporine	CYP3A4 Substrates	↑[Caspofungin].	Liver function monitoring
Tacrolimus	CYP3A4 Substrates	↓[Tacrolimus].	Monitoring of tacrolimus levels
Rifampicin, phenytoin	Enzyme induction	↑[Caspofungin].	Liver function monitoring

Updated guidelines recommend both fluconazole and an echinocandin for first-line treatment of non-neutropenic adults with candidemia or suspected systemic candidiasis. Although micafungin appears to be more effective than caspofungin in trial results, this cannot be extrapolated to anidulafungin. The IDSA guidelines favor the use of echinocandins for patients with moderate to severe disease, recent azole exposure, candidemia or suspected invasive candidiasis caused by *C. glabrata* or *C. krusei*. For the treatment of candidemia in neutropenic patients, the guidelines recommend first-line treatment with an echinocandin or lipid formulation of amphotericin B, and consider voriconazole as an alternative. For infections caused by *C. glabrata*, the use of an echinocandin or amphotericin B is preferred. (102).

For empirical treatment of invasive candidiasis in neutropenic patients, the guidelines recommend amphotericin B, voriconazole and caspofungin as first-line agents. Caspofungin is also indicated when invasive candidiasis is suspected in neutropenic patients and as salvage therapy in invasive aspergillosis (108).

For prophylaxis against *Candida* in HSCT patients, both micanfungin and fluconazole or posaconazole are recommended in HSCT patients with neutropenia. (108).

Echinocandins are well tolerated and have good safety profiles. The most frequent adverse effects can be hepatic alterations, such as hepatitis, hepatic failure, cutaneous rush, pruritus and facial reddening. (102).

5.3.3. Amphotericin B

Amphotericin B has activity against *Candida* and *Aspergillus* species, which, as we have already mentioned, are the most prevalent fungal pathogens in patients with neutropenia (Figure 11). (109)). Lipid formulations such as liposomal amphotericin B, amphotericin B lipid complex and amphotericin B colloidal dispersion are preferred to the classical amphotericin B formulations because of their lower nephrotoxicity (110). The traditional formulation (amphotericin B deoxycholate) is associated with adverse effects such as infusion reactions or even nephrotoxicity, which can lead to death. For this reason, several formulations of amphotericin B were developed in the 1990s to reduce its intrinsic toxicity, but at higher cost (111).

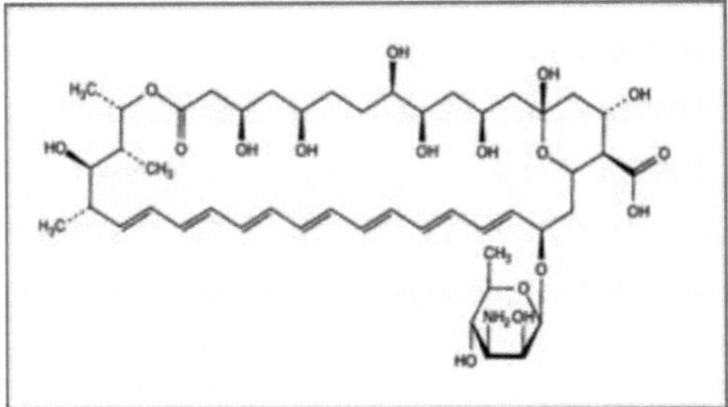

Figure 11. Chemical structure of amphotericin B (109).

Amphotericin B is a macrolide antifungal produced by the fungus *Streptomyces nodosus*. In the liposomal formulation, the lipophilic chain of amphotericin remains bound to the lipid bilayer of liposomes. This formulation contains a unilamellar lipid structure composed mostly of phosphatidylcholine, phosphatidylglycerol, and cholesterol (111).

The mechanism of action of amphotericin B is by drug binding to fungal membrane sterols. The result of this interaction is the alteration of membrane permeability resulting in the shedding of cellular contents. As a result, spillage of cellular contents and ultimately cell death occurs. There is a potential for toxicity in human cells due to binding of the drug to human cell membranes (112).

The formulation of amphotericin B as a lipid complex consists of a complex of amphotericin B with two phospholipids: L-α-dimyristoylphosphatidylcholine (DMPC) and L-α-dimyristoylphosphatidylglycerol (DMPG). The lipophilic moiety of amphotericin allows the drug molecules to form a curvilinear complex with the phospholipids.

The indications approved in Spain for the liposomal formulation are for the treatment of severe systemic mycoses, empirical treatment of mycoses in patients with severe neutropenia, as a consequence of hematological malignancies or due to the use of cytotoxic or immunosuppressive drugs, visceral leishmaniasis in immunocompetent and immunocompromised patients who have not responded to antimonials or conventional amphotericin B. One of the off-label uses of amphotericin B lipid complex is in a nebulized form as a prophylaxis measure in patients undergoing HSCT (59). This is because effective concentrations of nebulized amphotericin have been found to be effective in the respiratory tract (113). There are limited data on the usefulness of nebulized amphotericin as a single treatment for fungal infection, so it has been used as an adjuvant in combination with systemic voriconazole (114).

The most frequent adverse reactions observed in treatment with lipid complex amphotericin, according to the technical data sheet, were chills (15%), increased creatinine (13%), pyrexia (10%), nausea (7%) and vomiting (6%). In the case of treatment with the liposomal formulation, most patients experienced nephrotoxic effects, although according to double-blind trials, these are approximately half of those occurring with conventional amphotericin B or the lipid complex. The administration of amphotericin in any of its formulations frequently causes ionic disturbances such as hypokalemia, hyponatremia, hypomagnesemia, and hypocalcemia (115).

Unlike other antifungals mentioned, such as the azoles, amphotericin B does not show interactions at the cytochrome level, but its adverse effects can be worsened by the concomitant use of certain medications. The hypokalemia produced by the administration of amphotericin can cause cardiac alterations such as arrhythmias, especially with the concomitant use of digoxin; for this reason, special attention should be paid to the use of diuretics, laxatives and corticoids which can increase hypokalemia. (59). The administration of nephrotoxic medication can potentiate the nephrotoxic effect of amphotericin, which is why caution should be exercised when drugs such as iodinated contrast agents, aminoglycosides, platinum salts, methotrexate, foscarnet, antivirals and drugs widely used in HSCT patients such as cyclosporine and tacrolimus are used simultaneously (59).

The administration of nephroprotection protocols is recommended in those patients being treated with amphotericin B to avoid nephrotoxicity effects. Some strategies for renal protection are: correct hydration, administration of the drug in continuous infusion instead of rapid administrations, and adequate electrolyte replacement (115).

5.3.4.Trimethoprim and Sulfamethoxazole

Pneumocystis jirovecii is an opportunistic fungus that can cause pneumonia in immunocompromised patients. Timetoprim/sulfamethoxazole, also called cotrimoxazole association, is indicated in Spain for the treatment and prevention of pneumonia caused by Pneumocystis jiroveci, primary prophylaxis of toxoplasmosis, treatment of nocardiosis and melioidosis. (116) (Figure 12 and 13 (117) (118)).

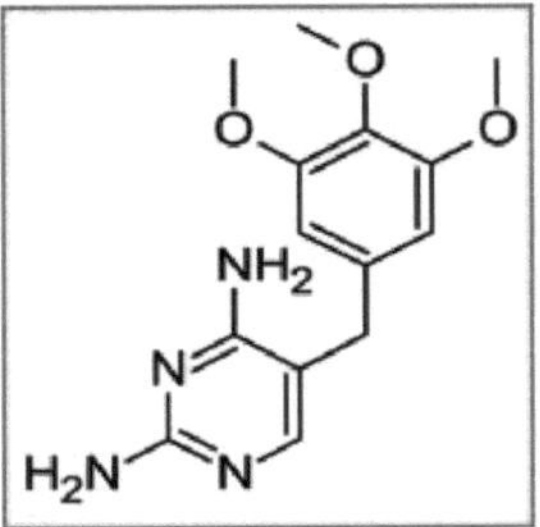

Figure 12. Chemical structure of trimethoprim (117)

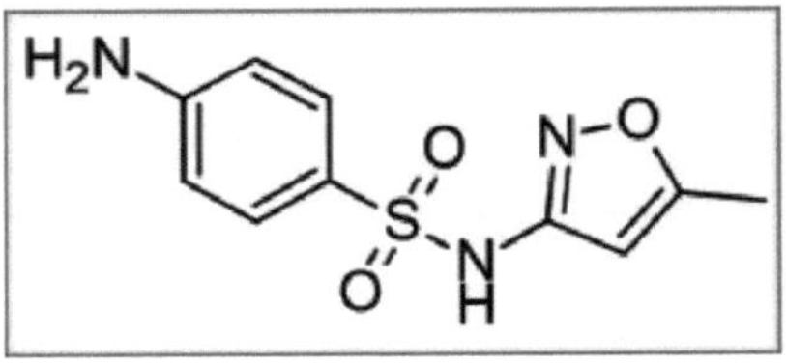

Figure 13. Chemical structure of sulfamethoxazole (118)

For the prophylaxis treatment of *Pneumocystis jirovecii* in HSCT patients, it should be administered 2 or 3 times per week and during the entire risk period (from engraftment to more than 6 months) and as long as immunosuppressants are being administered in the treatment.

The mechanism of action of sulfamethoxazole is bacteriostatic, which competitively blocks the utilization of para-aminobenzoic acid (PABA) for the production of bacterial cell dihydrofolate. Trimethoprim reversibly inhibits the bacterial dihydrofolate reductase (DHFR) enzyme involved in the folate metabolic pathway, which converts dihydrofolate to tetrahydrofolate. The combination of trimethoprim and sulfamethoxazole potentiates the activity marked in vitro and succeeds in blocking nucleic acid synthesis.

The mechanisms of resistance to sulfamethoxazole described are: a) the production of higher concentrations of PABA that displace sulfamethoxazole and reduce its inhibitory activity and b) production of altered dihydropteroate synthetase enzyme synthesized by plasmids, with reduced affinity for sulfamethoxazole. The most important resistance to trimethoprim is mediated by plasmids, through the production of the dihydrofolate reductase enzyme with reduced affinity for trimethoprim.

6. Conclusions

1. HSCT is a therapy to replace a damaged hematopoietic system with a healthy one from a donor. Hematopoietic stem cells are those capable of regenerating all cell types of blood cells.

2. Hematopoietic transplant patients undergo a process that predisposes them to various complications, such as toxicity caused by conditioning regimens, neutropenia, infections (bacterial, fungal or viral), transplant rejection or graft versus host disease.

3. *Aspergillus, Candida* and *Pneumocystis jirovecii* are the cause of 90% of invasive fungal infections in patients with hematologic diseases. The most frequent etiologic agent in these infections is *Aspergillus fumigatus.* The disease caused by this filamentous fungus is known as invasive aspergillosis.

4. The choice of prophylaxis for invasive fungal infection in the pre-graft phase is fluconazole, provided that the incidence of IFI by filamentous fungi is low. In places with a higher incidence, voriconazole or micafungin is considered as an alternative. In the post-grafting phase, the guidelines recommend the use of posaconazole.

5. Prophylaxis against *Candida* in hematopoietic stem cell transplant patients is recommended either micanfungin, fluconazole or posaconazole. *Pneumocystis jirovecii* prophylaxis with trimethoprim and oral sulfamethoxazole (cotrimoxazole) is the regimen of choice maintained from the graft for more than 6 months.

6. The empirical therapy that remains the standard of care in most centers is with caspofungin or liposomal amphotericin B. Targeted therapy for invasive aspergillosis is used in patients with proven fungal infection, for which voriconazole and isavuconazole are recommended. Liposomal amphotericin B is considered the alternative when azole drugs cannot be used due to intolerance problems, drug interactions, previous exposure to azole antifungals as prophylaxis and resistance problems.

7. Treatment of systemic candidiasis or candidemia with echinocandins is the first line of treatment, followed by targeted therapy once the *Candida* species and antifungal susceptibility are known. High-dose trimethoprim and sulfamethoxazole (co-trimoxazole) is the treatment of choice for those patients with *Pneumocystis jirovecii* infection. Amphotericin B formulations are the treatment of choice for mucormycosis.

8. Bibliography

Carreras E, Dufour C, Mohty M, Kröger N. The EBMT handbook: hematopoietic stem cell transplantation and cellular therapies. 2019.

Vogelsang GB, Hess AD. Graft-versus-host disease: new directions for a persistent problem. Blood. 1994;84(7):2061-7.

Simonin M, Dalissier A, Labopin M, Willasch A, Zecca M, Mouhab A, et al. More chronic GvHD and non-relapse mortality after peripheral blood stem cell compared with bone marrow in hematopoietic transplantation for paediatric acute lymphoblastic leukemia: a retrospective study on behalf of the EBMT Paediatric Diseases Working Party. Bone Marrow Transplantation. 2017;52(7):1071-3.

Dale DC, Cottle TE, Fier CJ, Bolyard AA, Bonilla MA, Boxer LA, et al. Severe chronic neutropenia: treatment and follow-up of patients in the Severe Chronic Neutropenia International Registry. American journal of hematology. 2003;72(2):82-93.

Freifeld AG, Bow EJ, Sepkowitz KA, Boeckh MJ, Ito JI, Mullen CA, et al. Clinical practice guideline for the use of antimicrobial agents in neutropenic patients with cancer: 2010 update by the Infectious Diseases Society of America. Clinical infectious diseases. 2011;52(4):e56-e93.

6. Kuderer NM, Dale DC, Crawford J, Cosler LE, Lyman GH. Mortality, morbidity, and cost associated with febrile neutropenia in adult cancer patients. Cancer. 2006;106(10):2258-66.

7. Carmona-Bayonas A, Jiménez-Fonseca P, Virizuela Echaburu J, Antonio M, Font C, Biosca M, et al. Prediction of serious complications in patients with seemingly stable febrile neutropenia: validation of the Clinical Index of Stable Febrile Neutropenia in a prospective cohort of patients from the FINITE study. Journal of Clinical Oncology. 2015;33(5):465-71.

Taplitz RA, Kennedy EB, Bow EJ, Crews J, Gleason C, Hawley DK, et al. Antimicrobial prophylaxis for adult patients with cancer-related immunosuppression: ASCO and IDSA clinical practice guideline update. Journal of Clinical Oncology. 2018;36(30):3043-54.

Flowers CR, Seidenfeld J, Bow EJ, Karten C, Gleason C, Hawley DK, et al. Antimicrobial prophylaxis and outpatient management of fever and neutropenia in adults treated for malignancy: American Society of Clinical Oncology clinical practice guideline. J Clin Oncol. 2013;31(6):794-810.

10. Taplitz RA, Kennedy EB, Bow EJ, Crews J, Gleason C, Hawley DK, et al. Outpatient management of fever and neutropenia in adults treated for malignancy: American Society of Clinical Oncology and Infectious Diseases Society of America Clinical Practice Guideline Update. J Clin Oncol. 2018;36(14):1443-53.

11. Cullen MH, Billingham LJ, Gaunt CH, Steven NM. Rational selection of patients for antibacterial prophylaxis after chemotherapy. Journal of clinical oncology. 2007;25(30):4821-8.

Bucaneve G, Micozzi A, Menichetti F, Martino P, Dionisi MS, Martinelli G, et al. Levofloxacin to prevent bacterial infection in patients with cancer and neutropenia. New England Journal of Medicine. 2005;353(10):977-87.

13. Beyar-Katz O, Dickstein Y, Borok S, Vidal L, Leibovici L, Paul M. Empirical antibiotics targeting Gram-positive bacteria for the treatment of febrile neutropenic patients with cancer. Cochrane Database of Systematic Reviews. 2017(6).

Maertens J, Theunissen K, Verhoef G, Verschakelen J, Lagrou K, Verbeken E, et al. Galactomannan and computed tomography-based preemptive antifungal therapy in neutropenic patients at high risk for invasive fungal infection: a prospective feasibility study. Clinical Infectious Diseases. 2005;41(9):1242-50.

Huang H, Li X, Zhu J, Ye S, Zhang H, Wang W, et al. Entecavir vs lamivudine for prevention of hepatitis B virus reactivation among patients with untreated diffuse large B-cell lymphoma receiving R-CHOP chemotherapy: a randomized clinical trial. Jama. 2014;312(23):2521-30.

Rubin LG, Levin MJ, Ljungman P, Davies EG, Avery R, Tomblyn M, et al. 2013 IDSA clinical practice guideline for vaccination of the immunocompromised host. Clinical infectious diseases. 2014;58(3):e44-e100.

Teshima T, Reddy P, Zeiser R. Reprint of: acute graft-versus-host disease: novel biological insights. Biology of Blood and Marrow Transplantation. 2016;22(3):S3-S8.

18. Masso J, Doy D. Prophylaxis and treatment of graft-versus-host disease in hematopoietic transplantation. The Hospital Pharmacist. 2001;119:32-7.

19. Grube M, Holler E, Weber D, Holler B, Herr W, Wolff D. Risk factors and outcome of chronic graft-versus-host disease after allogeneic stem cell transplantation-results from a single-center observational study. Biology of Blood and Marrow Transplantation. 2016;22(10):1781-91.

Cornell RF, Hari P, Drobyski WR. Engraftment syndrome after autologous stem cell transplantation: an update unifying the definition and management approach. Biology of Blood and Marrow Transplantation. 2015;21(12):2061-8.

21. Ruiz-Camps I, Jarque I. Invasive fungal disease by filamentous fungi in hematologic patients. Iberoamerican Journal of Mycology. 2014;31(4):249-54.

Girmenia C, Raiola AM, Piciocchi A, Algarotti A, Stanzani M, Cudillo L, et al. Incidence and outcome of invasive fungal diseases after allogeneic stem cell transplantation: a prospective study of the Gruppo Italiano Trapianto Midollo Osseo (GITMO). Biol Blood Marrow Transplant. 2014;20(6):872-80.

Cesaro S, Tridello G, Blijlevens N, Ljungman P, Craddock C, Michallet M, et al. Incidence, risk factors, and long-term outcome of acute leukemia patients with early candidemia after allogeneic stem cell transplantation: a study by the acute leukemia and infectious diseases working parties of European Society for Blood and Marrow Transplantation. Clinical Infectious Diseases. 2018;67(4):564-72.

24. Camps IR. Risk factors for invasive fungal infections in haematopoietic stem cell transplantation. Int J Antimicrob Agents. 2008;32 Suppl 2:S119-23.

Donnelly JP, Chen SC, Kauffman CA, Steinbach WJ, Baddley JW, Verweij PE, et al. Revision and Update of the Consensus Definitions of Invasive Fungal Disease From the European Organization for Research and Treatment of Cancer and the Mycoses Study Group Education and Research Consortium. Clin Infect Dis. 2020;71(6):1367-76.

26. Cadena J, Thompson GR, Patterson TF. Invasive aspergillosis: current strategies for diagnosis and management. Infectious Disease Clinics. 2016;30(1):125-42.

27. Mousavi B, Hedayati MT, Hedayati N, Ilkit M, Syedmousavi S. Aspergillus species in indoor environments and their possible occupational and public health hazards. Current medical mycology. 2016;2(1):36.

Ruhnke M, Kofla G, Otto K, Schwartz S. CNS aspergillosis. CNS drugs. 2007;21(8):659-76.

29. Nathan CL, Emmert BE, Nelson E, Berger JR. CNS fungal infections: A review. Journal of the neurological sciences. 2021;422:117325.

30. Shoham S, Levitz SM. The immune response to fungal infections. British journal of haematology. 2005;129(5):569-82.

31. Gottfredsson M, Perfect JR, editors. Fungal meningitis. Seminars in neurology; 2000: Copyright© 2000 by Thieme Medical Publishers, Inc., 333 Seventh Avenue, New ....

32. Maertens JA, Blennow O, Duarte RF, Munoz P. The current management landscape: aspergillosis. Journal of Antimicrobial Chemotherapy. 2016;71(suppl_2):ii23-ii9.

Maertens J, Cesaro S, Maschmeyer G, Einsele H, Donnelly JP, Alanio A, et al. ECIL guidelines for preventing Pneumocystis jirovecii pneumonia in patients with haematological malignancies and stem cell transplant recipients. Journal of Antimicrobial Chemotherapy. 2016;71(9):2397-404.

Stanzani M, Sassi C, Lewis RE, Tolomelli G, Bazzocchi A, Cavo M, et al. High resolution computed tomography angiography improves the radiographic diagnosis of invasive mold disease in patients with hematological malignancies. Clinical Infectious Diseases. 2015;60(11):1603-10.

35. Mylonakis E, Clancy CJ, Ostrosky-Zeichner L, Garey KW, Alangaden GJ, Vazquez JA, et al. T2 magnetic resonance assay for the rapid diagnosis of candidemia in whole blood: a clinical trial. Clinical Infectious Diseases. 2015;60(6):892-9.

36. Alanio A, Hauser PM, Lagrou K, Melchers WJ, Helweg-Larsen J, Matos O, et al. ECIL guidelines for the diagnosis of Pneumocystis jirovecii pneumonia in patients with haematological malignancies and stem cell transplant recipients. Journal of Antimicrobial Chemotherapy. 2016;71(9):2386-96.

37. Ullmann AJ, Lipton JH, Vesole DH, Chandrasekar P, Langston A, Tarantolo SR, et al. Posaconazole or fluconazole for prophylaxis in severe graft-versus-host disease. New England Journal of Medicine. 2007;356(4):335-47.

38. Girmenia C. Prophylaxis of invasive fungal diseases in patients with hematologic disorders. Haematologica. 2010;95(10):1630-2.

39. Garcia-Vidal C, Alastruey-Izquierdo A, Aguilar-Guisado M, Carratalà J, Castro C, Fernández-Ruiz M, et al. Executive summary of clinical practice guideline for the management of invasive diseases caused by Aspergillus: 2018 Update by the GEMICOMED-SEIMC/REIPI. Enferm Infecc Microbiol Clin (Engl Ed). 2019;37(8):535-41.

40. ECIL-5. The European Conference on Infections in Leukaemia 2013 [Available from: http://www.ecil-leukaemia.com.

41. Ruiz-Camps I, Aguado JM, Almirante B, Bouza E, Barbera CF, Len O, et al. Recommendations on the prevention of invasive fungal infection by filamentous fungi from the Spanish Society of Infectious Diseases and Clinical Microbiology (SEIMC). Infectious Diseases and Clinical Microbiology. 2010;28(3):172. e1-. e21.

Ruiz-Camps I, Aguado J, Almirante B, Bouza E, Ferrer-Barbera C, Len O, et al. Guidelines for the prevention of invasive mould diseases caused by filamentous fungi by the Spanish Society of Infectious Diseases and Clinical Microbiology (SEIMC). Clinical Microbiology and Infection. 2011;17:1-24.

43. Wang J, Zhou M, Xu JY, Zhou RF, Chen B, Wan Y. Comparison of Antifungal Prophylaxis Drugs in Patients With Hematological Disease or Undergoing Hematopoietic Stem Cell Transplantation: A Systematic Review and Network Meta-analysis. JAMA Netw Open. 2020;3(10):e2017652.

44. Stemler J, de Jonge N, Skoetz N, Sinkó J, Brüggemann RJ, Busca A, et al. Antifungal prophylaxis in adult patients with acute myeloid leukaemia treated with novel targeted therapies: a systematic review and expert consensus recommendation from the European Haematology Association. Lancet Haematol. 2022;9(5):e361-e73.

Robenshtok E, Gafter-Gvili A, Goldberg E, Weinberger M, Yeshurun M, Leibovici L, et al. Antifungal prophylaxis in cancer patients after chemotherapy or hematopoietic stem-cell transplantation: systematic review and meta-analysis. Database of Abstracts of Reviews of Effects (DARE): Quality-assessed Reviews [Internet]. 2007.

Blennow O, Remberger M, Klingspor L, Omazic B, Fransson K, Ljungman P, et al. Randomized PCR-based therapy and risk factors for invasive fungal infection following reduced-intensity conditioning and hematopoietic SCT. Bone marrow transplantation. 2010;45(12):1710-8.

47. Sun Y, Meng F, Han M, Zhang X, Yu L, Huang H, et al. Epidemiology, management, and outcome of invasive fungal disease in patients undergoing hematopoietic stem cell transplantation in China: a multicenter prospective observational study. Biology of Blood and Marrow Transplantation. 2015;21(6):1117-26.

48. Gøtzsche PC, Johansen HK. Routine versus selective antifungal administration for control of fungal infections in patients with cancer. Cochrane Database of systematic reviews. 2014(9).

49. Mercier T, Maertens J. Clinical considerations in the early treatment of invasive mould infections and disease. Journal of Antimicrobial Chemotherapy. 2017;72(suppl_1):i29-i38.

50. Tissot F, Agrawal S, Pagano L, Petrikkos G, Groll AH, Skiada A, et al. ECIL-6 guidelines for the treatment of invasive candidiasis, aspergillosis and mucormycosis in leukemia and hematopoietic stem cell transplant patients. haematologica. 2017;102(3):433.

51. Maertens JA, Raad II, Marr KA, Patterson TF, Kontoyiannis DP, Cornely OA, et al. Isavuconazole versus voriconazole for primary treatment of invasive mould disease caused by Aspergillus and other filamentous fungi (SECURE): a phase 3, randomised-controlled, non-inferiority trial. The Lancet. 2016;387(10020):760-9.

52. Marr KA, Schlamm HT, Herbrecht R, Rottinghaus ST, Bow EJ, Cornely OA, et al. Combination antifungal therapy for invasive aspergillosis: a randomized trial. Annals of internal medicine. 2015;162(2):81-9.

53. Resendiz Sharpe A, Lagrou K, Meis JF, Chowdhary A, Lockhart SR, Verweij PE, et al. Triazole resistance surveillance in Aspergillus fumigatus. Medical mycology. 2018;56(suppl_1):S83-S92.

54. Cornely O, Arikan-Akdagli S, Dannaoui E, Groll A, Lagrou K, Chakrabarti A, et al. ESCMID and ECMM joint clinical guidelines for the diagnosis and management of mucormycosis 2013. Clinical Microbiology and Infection. 2014;20:5-26.

Tortorano A, Richardson M, Roilides E, Van Diepeningen A, Caira M, Munoz P, et al. ESCMID and ECMM joint guidelines on diagnosis and management of hyalohyphomycosis: Fusarium spp, Scedosporium spp. and others. Clinical Microbiology and Infection. 2014;20:27-46.

Andes DR, Safdar N, Baddley JW, Playford G, Reboli AC, Rex JH, et al. Impact of treatment strategy on outcomes in patients with candidemia and other forms of invasive candidiasis: a patient-level quantitative review of randomized trials. Clinical infectious diseases. 2012;54(8):1110-22.

57. Lamoth F, Kontoyiannis DP. The Candida auris alert: facts and perspectives. The Journal of infectious diseases. 2018;217(4):516-20.

58. Maschmeyer G, Helweg-Larsen J, Pagano L, Robin C, Cordonnier C, Schellongowski P. ECIL guidelines for treatment of Pneumocystis jirovecii

pneumonia in non-HIV-infected haematology patients. Journal of Antimicrobial Chemotherapy. 2016;71(9):2405-13.

59. Nivoix Y, Ledoux MP, Herbrecht R. Antifungal Therapy: New and Evolving Therapies. Semin Respir Crit Care Med. 2020;41(1):158-74.

60. Pérez J, Guna R, Orta N, Gimeno C. New azoles: voriconazole. Quality control, Spanish Society of Infectious Diseases and Clinical Microbiology. 2003.

61. health Aedmyp. Voriconazole data sheet. 2019.

62. Marks DI, Pagliuca A, Kibbler CC, Glasmacher A, Heussel CP, Kantecki M, et al. Voriconazole versus itraconazole for antifungal prophylaxis following allogeneic haematopoietic stem-cell transplantation. British journal of haematology. 2011;155(3):318-27.

63. Levine MT, Chandrasekar PH. Adverse effects of voriconazole: over a decade of use. Clinical Transplantation. 2016;30(11):1377-86.

64. Owusu Obeng A, Egelund EF, Alsultan A, Peloquin CA, Johnson JA. CYP 2C19 Polymorphisms and Therapeutic Drug Monitoring of Voriconazole: Are We Ready for Clinical Implementation of Pharmacogenomics? Pharmacotherapy: The Journal of Human Pharmacology and Drug Therapy. 2014;34(7):703-18.

65. Moriyama B, Kadri S, Henning SA, Danner RL, Walsh TJ, Penzak SR. Therapeutic drug monitoring and genotypic screening in the clinical use of voriconazole. Current fungal infection reports. 2015;9(2):74-87.

66. Mori T, Aisa Y, Kato J, Nakamura Y, Ikeda Y, Okamoto S. Drug interaction between voriconazole and calcineurin inhibitors in allogeneic hematopoietic stem cell transplant recipients. Bone marrow transplantation. 2009;44(6):371-4.

67. Wang J-L, Chang C-H, Young-Xu Y, Chan KA. Systematic review and meta-analysis of the tolerability and hepatotoxicity of antifungals in empirical and definitive therapy for invasive fungal infection. Antimicrobial agents and chemotherapy. 2010;54(6):2409-19.

68. Saravolatz LD, Johnson LB, Kauffman CA. Voriconazole: a new triazole antifungal agent. Clinical infectious diseases. 2003;36(5):630-7.

69. Kwong WT, Hsu S. Pseudoporphyria associated with voriconazole. Journal of Drugs in Dermatology: JDD. 2007;6(10):1042-4.

70. Williams K, Mansh M, Chin-Hong P, Singer J, Arron ST. Voriconazole-associated cutaneous malignancy: a literature review on photocarcinogenesis in organ transplant recipients. Clinical infectious diseases. 2014;58(7):997-1002.

71. Brown JD, Lim L-l, Koning S. Voriconazole associated torsades de pointes in two adult patients with haematological malignancies. Medical mycology case reports. 2014;4:23-5.

72. Lustenberger DP, Granata JD, Scharschmidt TJ. Periostitis secondary to prolonged voriconazole therapy in a lung transplant recipient. Orthopedics. 2011;34(11):e793-e6.

73. Zonios DI, Banacloche JG, Childs R, Bennett JE. Hallucinations during voriconazole therapy. Clinical infectious diseases. 2008;47(1):e7-e10.

74. Baxter CG, Marshall A, Roberts M, Felton TW, Denning DW. Peripheral neuropathy in patients on long-term triazole antifungal therapy. Journal of antimicrobial chemotherapy. 2011;66(9):2136-9.

75. Luong M-L, Al-Dabbagh M, Groll AH, Racil Z, Nannya Y, Mitsani D, et al. Utility of voriconazole therapeutic drug monitoring: a meta-analysis. Journal of Antimicrobial Chemotherapy. 2016;71(7):1786-99.

76. Pascual A, Csajka C, Buclin T, Bolay S, Bille J, Calandra T, et al. Challenging recommended oral and intravenous voriconazole doses for improved efficacy and safety: population pharmacokinetics-based analysis of adult patients with invasive fungal infections. Clinical infectious diseases. 2012;55(3):381-90.

77. Herbrecht R, Denning DW, Patterson TF, Bennett JE, Greene RE, Oestmann J-W, et al. Voriconazole versus amphotericin B for primary therapy of invasive aspergillosis. New England Journal of Medicine. 2002;347(6):408-15.

78. Wikipedia. Isavuconazole 2019 [Chemical structure]. Available from: https://es.wikipedia.org/wiki/Isavuconazol.

79. Schmitt-Hoffmann A, Roos B, Heep M, Schleimer M, Weidekamm E, Brown T, et al. Single-ascending-dose pharmacokinetics and safety of the novel broad-spectrum antifungal triazole BAL4815 after intravenous infusions (50, 100, and 200 milligrams) and oral administrations (100, 200, and 400 milligrams) of its prodrug, BAL8557, in healthy volunteers. Antimicrobial agents and chemotherapy. 2006;50(1):279-85.

80. Cornely OA, Böhme A, Schmitt-Hoffmann A, Ullmann AJ. Safety and pharmacokinetics of isavuconazole as antifungal prophylaxis in acute myeloid leukemia patients with neutropenia: results of a phase 2, dose escalation study. Antimicrobial agents and chemotherapy. 2015;59(4):2078-85.

81. Jenks JD, Mehta SR, Hoenigl M. Broad spectrum triazoles for invasive mould infections in adults: which drug and when? Medical mycology. 2019;57(Supplement_2):S168-S78.

82. Falci DR, Pasqualotto AC. Profile of isavuconazole and its potential in the treatment of severe invasive fungal infections. Infection and drug resistance. 2013;6:163.

Marty FM, Ostrosky-Zeichner L, Cornely OA, Mullane KM, Perfect JR, Thompson III GR, et al. Isavuconazole treatment for mucormycosis: a single-arm open-label trial and case-control analysis. The Lancet infectious diseases. 2016;16(7):828-37.

84. Jenks JD, Salzer HJ, Prattes J, Krause R, Buchheidt D, Hoenigl M. Spotlight on isavuconazole in the treatment of invasive aspergillosis and mucormycosis: design, development, and place in therapy. Drug design, development and therapy. 2018;12:1033.

85. sanitary Aedmyp. Isavuconazole data sheet. 2021.

86. Miceli MH, Kauffman CA. Isavuconazole: a new broad-spectrum triazole antifungal agent. Clinical Infectious Diseases. 2015;61(10):1558-65.

Fontana L, Perlin DS, Zhao Y, Noble BN, Lewis JS, Strasfeld L, et al. Isavuconazole prophylaxis in patients with hematologic malignancies and hematopoietic cell transplant recipients. Clinical Infectious Diseases. 2020;70(5):723-30.

88. Stern A, Su Y, Lee YJ, Seo S, Shaffer B, Tamari R, et al. A single-center, open-label trial of isavuconazole prophylaxis against invasive fungal infection in patients undergoing allogeneic hematopoietic cell transplantation. Biology of Blood and Marrow Transplantation. 2020;26(6):1195-202.

89. Bowen CD, Tallman GB, Hakki M, Lewis Ⅱ JS. Isavuconazole to prevent invasive fungal infection in immunocompromised adults: initial experience at an academic medical centre. Mycoses. 2019;62(8):665-72.

90. Morris MI. Posaconazole: a new oral antifungal agent with an expanded spectrum of activity. American journal of health-system pharmacy. 2009;66(3):225-36.

91. health Aedmyp. Posaconazole tenica sheet 2019 [Available from: https://cima.aemps.es/cima/dochtml/ft/84010/FT_84010.html.

92. Schiller DS, Fung HB. Posaconazole: an extended-spectrum triazole antifungal agent. Clin Ther. 2007;29(9):1862-86.

93. Diekema D, Messer S, Hollis R, Jones R, Pfaller M. Activities of caspofungin, itraconazole, posaconazole, ravuconazole, voriconazole, and amphotericin B against 448 recent clinical isolates of filamentous fungi. Journal of Clinical Microbiology. 2003;41(8):3623-6.

94. Wong TY, Loo YS, Veettil SK, Wong PS, Divya G, Ching SM, et al. Efficacy and safety of posaconazole for the prevention of invasive fungal infections in immunocompromised patients: a systematic review with meta-analysis and trial sequential analysis. Sci Rep. 2020;10(1):14575.

95. Su H-C, Hua Y-M, Feng IJ, Wu H-C. Comparative effectiveness of antifungal agents in patients with hematopoietic stem cell transplantation: a systematic review and network meta-analysis. Infection and Drug Resistance. 2019;12:1311.

96. Kontoyiannis DP, Marr KA, Park BJ, Alexander BD, Anaissie EJ, Walsh TJ, et al. Prospective surveillance for invasive fungal infections in hematopoietic stem cell transplant recipients, 2001-2006: overview of the Transplant-Associated Infection Surveillance Network (TRANSNET) Database. Clinical Infectious Diseases. 2010;50(8):1091-100.

97. Wikipedia. Fluconazole 2021 [Chemical structure]. Available from: https://es.wikipedia.org/wiki/Fluconazol.

98. health Aedmyp. Fluconazole data sheet 2008 [Available from: https://cima.aemps.es/cima/dochtml/ft/65723/FichaTecnica_65723.html#5-propiedades-farmacol-gicas.

99. Wikipedia. Micafungin 2019 [Chemical structure]. Available from: https://es.wikipedia.org/wiki/Micafungina.

100. Wikipedia. Anidulafungin 2022 [Chemical structure]. Available from: https://en.wikipedia.org/wiki/Anidulafungin.

101. Wikipedia. Caspofungin 2020 [Chemical structure]. Available from: https://es.wikipedia.org/wiki/Caspofungina.

102. Sucher AJ, Chahine EB, Balcer HE. Echinocandins: the newest class of antifungals. Ann Pharmacother. 2009;43(10):1647-57.

103. Kim R, Khachikian D, Reboli AC. A comparative evaluation of properties and clinical efficacy of the echinocandins. Expert opinion on pharmacotherapy. 2007;8(10):1479-92.

104. Nakai T, Uno J, Ikeda F, Tawara S, Nishimura K, Miyaji M. In vitro antifungal activity of micafungin (FK463) against dimorphic fungi: comparison of yeast-like and mycelial forms. Antimicrobial Agents and Chemotherapy. 2003;47(4):1376-81.

105. Wiederhold NP, Lewis JS. The echinocandin micafungin: a review of the pharmacology, spectrum of activity, clinical efficacy and safety. Expert opinion on pharmacotherapy. 2007;8(8):1155-66.

106. Perlin DS. Resistance to echinocandin-class antifungal drugs. Drug Resistance Updates. 2007;10(3):121-30.

107. health Aedmyp. Caspofungin 2017 factsheet [Available from: https://cima.aemps.es/cima/dochtml/ft/81708/FichaTecnica_81708.html.

108. Pappas PG, Kauffman CA, Andes D, Benjamin Jr DK, Calandra TF, Edwards Jr JE, et al. Clinical practice guidelines for the management of candidiasis: 2009 update, from the Infectious Diseases Society of America. Clinical Infectious Diseases. 2009;48(5):503-37.

109. Wikipedia. Amphotericin B 2021 [Chemical structure]. Available from: https://es.wikipedia.org/wiki/Anfotericina_B.

110. Sandler ES, Mustafa MM, Tkaczewski I, Graham ML, Morrison VA, Green M, et al. Use of amphotericin B colloidal dispersion in children. Journal of pediatric hematology/oncology. 2000;22(3):242-6.

111. Steimbach LM, Tonin FS, Virtuoso S, Borba HH, Sanches AC, Wiens A, et al. Efficacy and safety of amphotericin B lipid-based formulations-A systematic review and meta-analysis. Mycoses. 2017;60(3):146-54.

112. health Aedmyp. Liposomal amphotericin B 2017 data sheet [Available from: https://cima.aemps.es/cima/dochtml/ft/61117/FT_61117.html#4-1-indicaciones-terap-uticas.

113. Husain S, Capitano B, Corcoran T, Studer SM, Crespo M, Johnson B, et al. Intrapulmonary disposition of amphotericin B after aerosolized delivery of amphotericin B lipid complex (Abelcet; ABLC) in lung transplant recipients. Transplantation. 2010;90(11):1215-9.

114. Gavaldà J, Meije Y, Fortún J, Roilides E, Saliba F, Lortholary O, et al. Invasive fungal infections in solid organ transplant recipients. Clinical Microbiology and infection. 2014;20:27-48.

115. Keane S, Geoghegan P, Povoa P, Nseir S, Rodriguez A, Martin-Loeches I. Systematic review on the first line treatment of amphotericin B in critically ill adults with candidemia or invasive candidiasis. Expert Review of Anti-infective Therapy. 2018;16(11):839-47.

116. sanitary Aedmyp. Fact sheet trimethoprim/sulfamethoxazole 2021 [Available from: https://cima.aemps.es/cima/pdfs/es/ft/48671/48671_ft.pdf.

117. Wikipedia. Trimethoprim 2021 [Chemical structure]. Available from: https://es.wikipedia.org/wiki/Trimetoprima.

118. Wikipedia. Sulfamethoxazole 2021 [Chemical structure]. Available from: https://es.wikipedia.org/wiki/Sulfametoxazol.

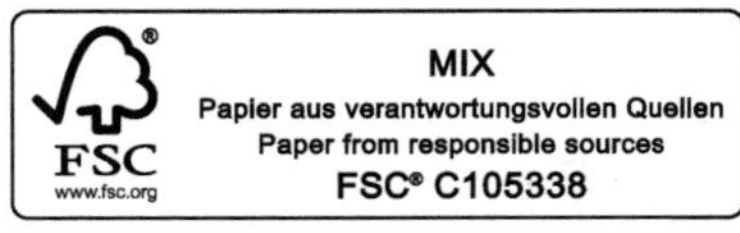

Printed by Books on Demand GmbH, Norderstedt / Germany